FEMALE
BRAIN
GONE
INSANE

FEMALE BRAIN GONE INSANE

An Emergency Guide for Women
Who Feel like They Are
Falling Apart

MIA LUNDIN, R.N.C., N.P.

Health Communications, Inc.
Deerfield Beach, Florida

www.hcibooks.com

DISCLAIMER: This book is not intended as a substitute for the advice and/or medical care of the reader's physician, nor is it meant to discourage or dissuade the reader from the advice of his or her physician. The reader should regularly consult with a physician in matters relating to his or her health, and especially with regard to symptoms that may require diagnosis. Any eating or lifestyle regimen should be undertaken under the direct supervision of the reader's physician. Moreover, anyone with chronic or serious ailments should undertake any eating and lifestyle program, and/or changes to his or her personal eating and lifestyle regimen, under the direct supervision of his or her physician. If the reader has any questions concerning the information presented in this book, or its application to his or her particular medical profile, or if the reader has unusual medical or nutritional needs or constraints that may conflict with the advice in this book, he or she should consult his or her physician. If the reader is pregnant or nursing she should consult her physician before embarking on the nutrition and lifestyle program outlined in this book. The reader should not stop prescription medications without the advice and guidance of his or her personal physician.

Library of Congress Cataloging-in-Publication Data

Lundin, Mia.
    Female brain gone insane : an emergency guide for women who feel like they are falling apart / by Mia Lundin.
      p. cm.
    Includes bibliographical references and index.
    ISBN-13: 978-0-7573-1416-2
    ISBN-10: 0-7573-1416-3
    1. Women—Psychology. I. Title.
    HQ1206.L865 2009
    155.6'33—dc22

                                    2009025616

Publisher: Health Communications, Inc.
            3201 S.W. 15th Street
            Deerfield Beach, FL 33442–8190

Cover design by Larissa Hise Henoch
Interior design and formatting by Lawna Patterson Oldfield

*This book is dedicated to
all the women who felt like they were
going insane and suffered in silence
or without appropriate help
or explanations.*

Contents

Part Three: Supplementary Steps for Adrenal and Thyroid Support

Acknowledgments

TO MY MOTHER, BRITT LUNDIN, and in memory of my father, Arne Lundin, who always let me do what I was set to do, and who did not complain when I had to leave my country to walk my path.

To my oldest and very intelligent son, Emil, who as a seven-year-old boy got uprooted and accompanied me on my journey. It was hard for him, but he has never complained.

To my sweet son William, who came into this world to give me the experience of postpartum depression so I could understand what feeling insane felt like and whose beautiful singing I listen to when I need comfort.

To my independent daughter, Amanda, who has watched me patiently at the computer, writing on my book day and night while writing her own amazing poetry.

To my best friends Ewy Axelsson and Yvonne Ebberoth, who love me unconditionally and support me in all my endeavors.

To Ilene Segalove, who helped me write this book. Without her witty and artistic brain all the information would still just be swirling in my head.

To my agent, Gareth Esersky, at Carol Mann Agency, who sold the book to Health Communications, Inc.

To Michele Matrisciani at HCI, who believed in the book and convinced the rest of the board to acquire it.

To Ann Gossy, who helped me edit the book so you all would really get what I wrote.

To all my wonderful patients, who have trusted me in their health care and told many other women to do the same. They have all taught me a lot of what I know.

To Areli Contreras, my receptionist and medical assistant, who can multitask like no one else while still keeping a smile on her face. I would not be able to run a practice without her help.

And at last but not least, to Abbey, my dog, who patiently sat at my feet waiting for a walk while I was lost in my creation of writing this book.

I am so grateful to all of you.

Preface:
My Female Brain Gone Insane

IN 1990, WHEN I WAS THIRTY-FOUR YEARS OLD, I gave birth
to my second child and settled into being a happy and contented mom.
After five months of successful and gratifying nursing, I decided to
wean my son. He went easily from breast to bottle, but I didn't. All of a
sudden, I began to experience horrible feelings I had never known
before. Waves of nervousness and anxiety rushed through my body. I
couldn't control the overwhelming sensations of fear and panic. I could
not sleep. I was unable to eat. I felt like I was spinning out of control. I
had no idea where this was coming from, and I was convinced I was
going insane. Why else would I feel this way? I'd always been a secure
and confident person and, when I weaned my first son, years before, I
was just fine. In six short weeks, I lost twenty pounds and with it, total
control over my own emotions. I also lost the hope of ever getting back
to normal. I wondered, *What was wrong with me? Was I falling apart?*

In an attempt to maintain some sanity, I began an avid search to find
out what was going on. There wasn't much written about my specific
symptoms (this was years before Brooke Shields's book and others on
the subject of postpartum depression). I finally discovered the writings
of an English doctor named Katarina Dalton who identified suffering

like mine as a type of postpartum depression (PPD). Dr. Dalton successfully treated women suffering from PPD and premenstrual syndrome (PMS) with pills, vaginal suppositories, and injections of natural
micronized progesterone. I began to feel some hope.

At the time, I was working as a nurse practitioner in a gynecologist's
office in Los Angeles. In spite of my daily freaking out, I had the where-
withal and was desperate enough to try out Dr. Dalton's protocol. I
asked my supervising doctor to give me a shot of natural progesterone.
Within twenty minutes, all my symptoms: the anxiety, the fear, and
panic simply disappeared! Sadly, the effect lasted only about forty-eight
hours. I tried another shot and had the same remarkable relief. Since I
wasn't really clear or confident about what I was doing, I stopped the
progesterone shots and sought psychiatric help. The doctor confirmed
my diagnosis of postpartum depression and gave me a now antiquated
tricyclic antidepressant. Apprehensive about the pills, I was reluctant
to take them, but after about two months I consented. Although I never
felt quite right on the medication, I began to improve little by little, and
in about a year, I recovered from PPD and the trauma of losing control.
Although almost nineteen years have now passed, I will never forget
what it was like to suffer from my female brain gone insane.

My own experience with postpartum depression and the relief of my
symptoms—thanks to the injections of natural progesterone—fed my
curiosity about the intricate dance between female hormones and the
female brain. I also knew I wanted to find ways to help women handle
the emotional meltdown associated with hormone imbalances in the
most natural ways possible. After my own recovery, I began work as a
nurse practitioner at a women's clinic in Manhattan Beach, California.
At the time (now it feels like ancient history), menopausal women were
given estrogen such as Premarin, primarily to eliminate symptoms of

night sweats and hot flashes as well as to prevent osteoporosis.

As its name implies, *Pre-mar-in* is derived from the urine of pregnant mares; a cocktail of estrogens that are natural to horses, not women! It is probably a great natural treatment for menopause if you have four hooves and a tail, but obviously, we do not! Premarin was often prescribed in combination with Provera, a synthetic progesterone that belongs more in a science lab than in a woman's body. This protocol made absolutely no sense, especially since there are plant-based bioidentical hormones available that look and behave identically to our own. I started to switch my patient's hormones from the horse estrogen and synthetic progesterone to the bioidentical ones. Almost immediately, changes in so many women's symptoms, personality, and quality of life were positive and remarkable. And, it was only much later that I realized hormone treatment was just part of the equation to help women find their balance.

Today, I know that women do better on bioidentical hormones. Why? The molecules of the hormones in bioidentical hormone replacement therapy look identical to the hormones the ovaries produce. Both estrogen in bioidentical hormone replacement therapy and estrogen produced by the ovaries function as one of the brain's natural antidepressants by supporting healthy levels of serotonin and other neurotransmitters in the female brain. Today, I also know we can boost a woman's brain chemistry with nutritional supplements such as amino acids and certain vitamins to levels where it produces feelings of well-being and peacefulness. **Bioidentical hormones plus natural brain chemistry precursors equal the new working formula for sanity and contentment.**

In 1995, I gave birth to my third child, a beautiful daughter. This time I was better prepared for the warning signs of a possible postpartum depression. Armed with knowledge of what hormones and nutritional supplements to take and a great support team consisting of a gynecologist who believed in bioidentical hormones and a great psychologist, I sailed through postpartum without much suffering. Today, I am the owner, founder, and director of The Center for Hormonal and Nutritional Balance, Inc., in Santa Barbara, California, where I apply my Female Brain Gone Insane experience to help thousands of female patients who suffer emotionally from the result of hormonal and neurotransmitter (brain chemistry) imbalances get back on the road to health and happiness.

I practice what is called functional medicine, a science-based health care approach that assesses and treats underlying causes of illness through individually tailored therapies to restore health and improve the function of the body. When I see a woman for the first time, we spend almost two hours together and talk a lot. I diligently listen so that I can really hear and understand how my patient feels and find out all I can about the specific problems she struggles to handle. You'll meet some of my patients and read their stories and successful outcomes throughout *Female Brain Gone Insane*. Naturally, when I see a patient, I take a complete history, do a physical exam, and review test results (saliva, urine, and blood) to determine what type of imbalance affects each woman. I use a combination of holistic approaches to analyze and treat interdependent systems of the body to create a dynamic balance integral for good health.

Traditional medicine tends to mask symptoms. I search for and identify the underlying causes of symptoms. Women tell me about their anxiety, irritability, brain fog, erratic weeping, and more. Their symptoms speak volumes and tell me how their bodies and brain chemistry are out of balance. I, in turn, provide their bodies with what they scream for, which includes bioidentical hormones, as well as supplements, brain-mood food, sometimes adrenal and thyroid support, and lifestyle changes that help repair and rebalance. Then the body's natural intelligence can take care of the rest.

I am often a woman's "last-hope" practitioner. Women who come see me have already met with all kinds of specialists from gynecologists to urologists, from neurologists to psychiatrists. They sit across my desk and share how frightened and desperate they feel. They ask, *Will I ever get well?* or *Will I ever feel at peace again?* They tell me how their doctors prescribed everything from birth control pills to antidepressants and bipolar medication, but nothing made them feel like themselves. Some are nearly suicidal, others live in the depths of overflowing sadness, and some are plain exhausted, while others are hopeless or spinning in so much anxiety they can barely speak. No matter their condition, they share their deep frustration from not getting answers to their questions and not having their health needs met. Most women know there is something radically wrong and tell me they deserve better. I am honored to have been there for them and to have helped make a positive difference in their lives.

I know it's difficult to consider yet another set of options and solutions. Your brain might not be operating at its optimum level right now, and plowing through another book on women and hormones is not what you want to do. However, I promise you, I have made every effort to make *Female Brain Gone Insane* as simple and easy to use as possible. It is designed as your own hands-on how-to manual back to health. Think of it as a long consultation with me, a virtual meeting of sorts, one that gives you the tools, recommendations, and empowerment to take care of yourself. Right now.

Strange as it may seem, I couldn't be more grateful for the lessons I learned from my own female brain gone insane. After all of these years,

I still remember vividly what an emotional meltdown feels like. I know the ravages of riding the radical ups and downs of hormonal change, thinking it will never end. I also know how overwhelmed, lost, and desperate you can feel if you suffer alone. So join me as I share the wisdom I have gathered, along with profiles of women who have gone through my treatment program and are living happy, healthy lives. Knowledge is power, and I promise, the more you listen to, understand, and learn how to feed your body what it actually screams for, the faster you will regain control over your emotional ups and downs and physical discomfort and heal. May this book provide you with the information, inspiration, and support to pull yourself out of the trenches where you feel like you are falling apart and bring you to safe ground. Reclaim the feeling of balance and harmony that allows you to live the rest of your life to its fullest.

Introduction

ARE YOU ON AN EMOTIONAL ROLLER COASTER? Do you feel like you are losing it or going insane? One minute you are agitated and lash out irrationally at friends and loved ones. The next minute you weep and want to be held. You feel overwhelmed, sad beyond words, or scared for no apparent reason. You find it difficult to shut down your anxious brain to go to sleep and then you wake in the middle of the night wide-eyed, with your heart racing. You push forward with all of your might, but inside you feel like you are falling apart. You are not alone. Many women feel just like you, hoping and praying for an end to their suffering.

All women share the same desires. We want to make life run smoothly for those we love. We spend our days fulfilling endless commitments and are dedicated to take care of everyone else's needs. But we can only do so much. Exhausted because we try to achieve impossibly high standards, we rush around to keep full schedules and make sure everyone is cared for. What happens? We rarely rest or pay attention to what is going on inside of us. In our mid-thirties to late-fifties, our bodies go through many changes. Our hormones, particularly the female hormone estrogen, can fluctuate radically, and our brain chemistry can become imbalanced. Having too much or too little of the hormones and neurotransmitters required for health and balance can create all kinds of symptoms that make us feel out of sorts, or worse. Common symptoms include crying spells, irritability, rage, panic attacks, uncontrolled irrational tantrums, anxiety, depression, faulty memory, insomnia, confusion, and fuzzy brains. Over time, we forget the happy, functional person we once were, and we only see ourselves as miserable with this litany of discomforts. Riding an emotional roller coaster is consuming and debilitating, plus it can be just plain terrifying.

Meet Jen

Jen was shaky and looked worn out as she sat down across from me, cradling the Kleenex box in her arms. She burst into tears and said, "I feel like a complete failure." Jen's best friend, Gloria, who accompanied her, confessed she was alarmed at Jen's erratic behavior including her deep fear of being alone. Gloria wrapped her arm around her friend's trembling shoulders. Then, Jen told me she worried that this nightmare might never end.

I asked her to tell me how she felt. "My brain is racing all the time. I can't seem to relax. I have a tough time falling asleep and bolt straight up in bed, wide awake every hour or two with a pounding heart. I feel like an elephant is sitting on my chest, and I can barely breathe. I also seem to be filled with rage and snap at everyone and everything. To be honest, I cannot stand myself or my life anymore," Jen broke down and apologized for her tears. "I have been agitated and anxious for at least three or four months, and I don't know what to do. I feel completely lost. Mia, I am afraid I'm falling apart."

I asked more questions. Jen informed me that in the last six months her periods were much heavier and more frequent than her usual twenty-eight day cycle. Based on Jen's symptoms, I knew she was in the hormonal phase called perimenopause. Her symptoms also pointed to a deficiency of the feel-good brain neurotransmitter known as serotonin. I ordered a urine test to measure Jen's brain chemistry levels, and it revealed she lacked enough serotonin. I started Jen on bioidentical progesterone, my basic vitamin supplement program, a protein shake with breakfast, and a precursor to serotonin called 5-HTP to raise her serotonin level.

Jen called me two weeks later, well before our scheduled one-month follow-up. She sounded like a new person. She slept through the night and was no longer wracked with anxiety or agitation. Within two months of following my plan, her periods had normalized back to twenty-eight day cycles, and she felt like her old self again.

Jen suffered from what I call Female Brain Gone Insane. Yes, it's a bit of a dramatic title, but over the last two decades, I've treated many women who feel exactly this way. Female Brain Gone Insane involves a disruption in the intimate dance between female hormones and brain chemistry, which results in deeply discordant emotional symptoms and endless distress. Women tell me they are falling apart and I believe them. Why? As with Jen, their symptoms are real, and they are caused by a true neurological brain-endocrine hormone imbalance. With just the right treatment, Jen was able to get through it. You will too!

Female Brain Gone Insane, inspired by my female patients, brings together the most current research, protocols, tips, and powerfully effective solutions I've collected and crafted from many years of listening to and helping women regain emotional control, balance, and well-being. It takes everything I've learned and distills all of it into a practical emergency guidebook that leads you through an easy-to-follow customized Emotional Rescue Plan guaranteed to alleviate your current emotional distress. It would be great if you didn't have to work, if you didn't have a mortgage to pay or kids and aging parents to take care of; but you do, and you can't make those external stressors go away. However, simple hormone and brain chemistry adjustments can help "thicken your skin," and "lengthen your fuse," to change the way you perceive and react to physical and emotional stress. You are not defective, but rather a wonderful and sensitive woman who will feel good and thrive again. *Female Brain Gone Insane* will get you back on the road to sanity in no time.

The Hormone-Brain Connection

There are legitimate reasons you feel the way you do. Current scientific research, epidemiological studies, and clinical trials clarify and prove a real and profound interaction between your hormones and brain chemistry that can create a set of symptoms and an emotional state that make you feel, well, insane. We now know that the brain and its many neurotransmitters are highly dependent on estrogen. When estrogen levels shift or become erratic, women experience emotional ups and downs, insomnia, and other cognitive disruptions such as brain fog and memory loss. Endocrinologists now understand that women are not only vulnerable to emotional upsets when they are premenstrual, but they are vulnerable during all of the reproductive turning points in their lives, including after childbirth and during perimenopause and menopause, when hormones and brain chemistry fluctuate the most. When you add the stressors of daily life to the mix, the imbalances become amplified and women suffer.

I've treated many women who were stuck in the stressful loop of our twenty-first century lifestyle. Haven't you wanted to be the best mom, wife, partner, or coworker but found yourself in the middle of a chaotic world, overloaded and spinning too fast or so wiped out you could not get off the couch? No longer able to put up with the daily stressors of life, have you struggled to salvage what was left of yourself and your relationships? Do you feel life may never be normal, let alone happy again? You may have no idea what to do, where to turn, or how to save yourself, so you get busy. You cram exercise into an impossibly packed schedule. You clean the house, organize the closets, and try to keep things straight. But, no matter what you do, you find no peace, no joy, and no ease. You may even look around and think other women somehow have it made, while you feel odd, different, and frankly, weird. Not wanting to share how out of sorts you feel, you keep your suffering to yourself. Filled with doubt and a deep sense of failure you ask yourself, *Will I ever feel like me again?*

Regardless of job description or pay scale, all of us juggle multiple roles as workers, moms, daughters, sisters, wives, and homemakers. Our hands are full with difficult teenagers, aging parents, and tense spouses. We have to deal with problems at work, traffic jams, and normal routines like going to the grocery store and innumerable other errands. While we run around doing too much, our bodies show stress and we experience a litany of unpleasant symptoms. And, we rarely pay attention to them. Our innate intelligence shouts out, *Hey, you! Slow down. Breathe. Relax. When was the last time you had a good night's sleep and a nutritional meal?* And what do you do with that endless stream of intuitive knowing that tries so hard to interrupt the rat race? Maybe you slip into a yoga class to stretch for a quick hour, but then you're off to gulp another cup of coffee and dash back into your demanding life. Maybe you sit down for a glass of wine and kick off your shoes. But do these temporary distractions and activities really bring you lasting peace or calm? Probably not.

There Is a Solution

Many health care practitioners still fail to recognize the connection between women's hormones and their mental states. Obliged to offer some panacea, they do their best to address your condition and pre-scribe blood pressure medications, antidepressants, or sleeping pills. Possibly, your gynecologist has offered you birth control pills in an attempt to "normalize" your hormones, or a psychiatrist has suggested antidepressants to "normalize" your brain chemistry. These so-called treatments may not work at all, they may give some relief, or they may leave you with unpleasant side effects.

Sadly, you may feel as though your health care practitioner didn't hear you or failed to treat what is really going on. Too many women are told, "Your emotional suffering is all in your head." Your doctor may say your symptoms are caused by stress, without providing any suggestions of what to do or what to take in order to feel better. Neither birth con-trol pills nor antidepressants will treat the true underlying problem, which is a hormone-brain chemistry imbalance. The birth control pill, a combination of synthetic estrogen and synthetic progesterone, can actually shut down the production of your own natural hormones, which explains why emotional symptoms often worsen when some women start taking them. The serotonin reuptake inhibitor (SSRI) anti-depressants such as Prozac, Lexapro, and Celexa do not increase the level of serotonin, but rather recycle whatever serotonin is already in your brain. If your brain produces little or no serotonin to begin with—the drugs won't have enough to recycle, so they won't do much good.

In truth, these prescription medications do not address the source of the hormone-brain chemistry imbalance and, therefore, may not bring relief. Nor will you find the answers in a health food store where you'll likely scour the miles of women's health shelves and end up taking advice from a young, newly employed store clerk who will try to sell you a combination of St. John's wort, black cohosh, dong quai, and soy flavinoids with hope-inspiring names like Soy Joy and Revival Soy. Don't buy into it.

Here's what you need to know. You are not suffering from a deficiency that can be remedied by St. John's wort, black cohosh, dong quai, or soy. These preparations cannot alleviate your symptoms and cure you. Your own daily or accumulated life stressors coupled with an imbalance in your brain chemistry and hormones cause your symptoms. And your symptoms scream for the correct nutrients in the form of hormones, supplements, and brain-mood foods to get you feeling right again.

Consider this analogy. When you drive your car and the oil light turns red, I am sure you don't smash the light with a hammer and continue driving. And you don't add orange juice to your engine instead of oil, do you? Rather, you identify the specific problem: your car needs oil. You take it in for service, or put the oil in yourself, so the engine won't die.

In many ways, your body is just like your car. It is, obviously, a higher functioning, intelligent piece of machinery, but it needs the right kind of fuel to function. Consider that your emotional and physical symptoms are like the bright red oil light glowing on your dashboard. When you feel exhausted, anxious, deeply sad, or plain uneasy, your body and brain require the appropriate raw material—in the form of bioidentical hormones—to mimic the brain chemicals and hormones the body used to make all by itself. It is actually very simple to restore balance once you have the information, guidelines, and appropriate ingredients in place. And this book provides you with everything you need.

In Part One: The Science Behind the Insanity and the Solution, you'll find out more about the science behind why you feel like you do. You'll also get a better understanding of what bioidentical hormones are and why they are so effective and safe in helping you find balance.

Part Two: Four Steps to Sanity—Your Emotional Rescue Plan helps you identify your current hormonal phase. You will also determine your emotional type, known as your brain chemistry profile. You'll find out if you are the Revved Up and Anxious Type, the I Can't Get Off the Couch Type, or the Combination Type. Once you pin point your hormonal phase and emotional type, you'll gain insight about yourself and will be able fill in Your Emotional Rescue Plan with ease and confidence. You'll also learn what essential brain-mood foods, supplements, and hormones you'll need to get your body back into balance.

Part Three: Supplemental Steps for Adrenal and Thyroid Support will teach you about your adrenal and thyroid glands and offer the appropriate medical tests to determine if you would benefit from additional support for these glands.

I promise you, the emotional roller coaster will stop, and it won't take long. Take a deep breath and relax a little. With this book in hand, you are well on your way to regaining your health and happiness. Let's get started!

How to Use This Book

THIS BOOK IS DESIGNED TO GET YOU feeling better as quickly as possible. You must put your own well-being first, so you need an easy way to find out exactly what to do for your own particular situation. Although everyone is different, we all share the same basic body-mind make up. No matter how old you are or what you've been through, you can take charge of your insane female brain. *Female Brain Gone Insane* doesn't dwell on psychological probing to find out why you feel like you are falling apart. Let's just agree: your hormones and brain chemistry are out of balance! Once you identify your symptoms, hormonal phase, and emotional type you will know where you stand and what to do to feel good again.

- Read Part One: The Science Behind the Insanity to gain a full understanding of bioidentical hormones and how your brain works. If you feel overwhelmed, extremely sad, or anxious and are having a difficult time concentrating on reading and absorbing information, feel free to skip Part One and immediately get started with Part Two.
- Begin Part Two: Four Steps to Sanity—Your Emotional Rescue Plan and take action to start feeling better today. Make a copy of:
  - Your Monthly Symptom Tracker (pages 13–14)

• Your Emotional Rescue Plan (pages 15–21)

You can download the forms at www. femalebraingoneinsane.com. Then:

• Fill in the Monthly Symptom Tracker on a daily basis for one month before you begin or use it as you start your program and chart your progress as your symptoms diminish.
• Follow Steps One, Two, Three, and Four. You will quickly identify your hormonal phase and emotional type along with just the right bioidentical hormones, nutritional supplements, brain-mood foods, and lifestyle changes you need.
• Fill in the Emotional Rescue Plan form to create a plan tailored to your unique needs.
• If you like, read and follow the directions in Steps Five and Six to learn more about your adrenal and thyroid glands. Then take the appropriate medical tests to determine if you would benefit from additional support for these glands.
• Make sure to read the Afterword: Staying Sane—How to Maintain Emotional Balance for Life to maintain your balance and serenity.
• Read the Resources section at the end of the book for more ideas, information, tests, and useful websites.

Your Monthly Symptom Tracker

Your symptoms are the key to figuring out what is going on inside your body and mind. Blood, saliva, and urine tests may help identify your hormone and brain chemical levels, but how you feel right now is what really counts. I will suggest some tests you can take later on if you like, but there is a lot you can do right now without sending away for lab kits or even visiting your doctor.

Use the Monthly Symptom Tracker as a tool to help you keep track of what you feel on a daily basis. It allows you to see patterns—the ups and downs of your emotional state—throughout the month. Your symptoms speak, so it is important to listen to them. They will help you identify your current hormonal phase and emotional type, so you can begin to build your Emotional Rescue Plan.

Refer to your Monthly Symptom Tracker every day and place an X next to each symptom you experience. Choose from mild, moderate, severe, or none—depending on how intense each symptom seems to you. Indicate when you have your period on the menstruation line by placing an X on the appropriate days.

Here are the most common symptoms I see in my practice because of imbalanced brain chemistry.

- Feeling anxious or panicky (intense feelings of fear or uneasiness)
- Crying spells (crying more than normally)
- Feeling depressed (feelings of sadness, gloom, and inadequacy)
- Feeling "flat" (emotionless)
- Rapid thoughts (mind doesn't seem to be able to shut down)
- Lack of alertness (difficulty focusing, concentrating, or remembering things)
- Insomnia (not able to fall asleep or waking up in the middle of night)
- Irritability (feeling "cranky")
- Rage (feeling of intense anger)
- Lack of motivation (not able to get anything done)
- Feeling overwhelmed (life and daily tasks seem to be too much for you to handle)
- Feeling withdrawn (you tend to want to be alone)

When I review these symptoms with my patients, I learn a great deal about what might be going on with their hormones, including the female hormones, estrogen and progesterone, as well as the adrenal and thyroid hormones. I also get a good read on what is going on with their brain chemistry, particularly the levels and imbalances of the neuro-transmitters. (More on this later. Just know that too much or too little of important neurotransmitters can create emotional unease.) Lab tests also clarify what is going on inside the body, and I believe these tests are valuable. But in *Female Brain Gone Insane,* you will learn how to listen to and identify your own symptoms so you can get started immediately and take tangible action steps toward sanity.

✓ Your Monthly Symptom Tracker

Month: _____   Your Name: _____

Day of the Month		1	2	3	4	5	6	7	8	9	10	11	12	13	14	15	16	17	18	19	20	21	22	23	24	25	26	27	28	29	30	31
Menstruation																																
Feeling anxious or panicky	severe																															
	moderate																															
	mild																															
	none																															
Crying spells	severe																															
	moderate																															
	mild																															
	none																															
Feeling depressed	severe																															
	moderate																															
	mild																															
	none																															
Feeling "flat"	severe																															
	moderate																															
	mild																															
	none																															
Rapid thoughts	severe																															
	moderate																															
	mild																															
	none																															
Lack of alertness	severe																															
	moderate																															
	mild																															
	none																															

Continue on next page

✓ Your Monthly Symptom Tracker (Continued)

Month: _____   Your Name: _____

Day of the Month		1	2	3	4	5	6	7	8	9	10	11	12	13	14	15	16	17	18	19	20	21	22	23	24	25	26	27	28	29	30	31
Menstruation																																
Insomnia	severe																															
	moderate																															
	mild																															
	none																															
Irritability	severe																															
	moderate																															
	mild																															
	none																															
Rage	severe																															
	moderate																															
	mild																															
	none																															
Lack of motivation	severe																															
	moderate																															
	mild																															
	none																															
Feeling overwhelmed	severe																															
	moderate																															
	mild																															
	none																															
Feeling withdrawn	severe																															
	moderate																															
	mild																															
	none																															

Design Your Emotional Rescue Plan

Use the worksheet below to record the Emotional Rescue Plan tailored to your unique situation. Each step corresponds to a chapter in the book. And each chapter will tell you precisely what to fill in on your worksheet. You will learn the exact hormones, nutritional supplements, foods, and lifestyle changes you need to break out of your discomfort and launch into an emotionally stable, satisfying, and healthy life.

Your Emotional Rescue Plan Worksheet

Name: _____   Date: _____

Work through each step by reading the chapter in the book that corresponds to it. As you read, you will be able to identify with other women's stories and their symptoms. Take the action recommended for your profile and record it here. Remember, you only need to finish Steps One through Four to benefit from the program.

Step One: Identify Your Hormonal Phase
Read pages: 67–99
Are you: ❏ Normal ❏ PMS ❏ Perimenopause ❏ Menopause ❏ Hysterectomy

My Hormonal Phase is: _____

Treatment:
Bioidentical hormones (if any) recommended based on my phase:
1. _____
2. _____
3. _____

What to ask my doctor:
1. Request the prescription bioidentical hormones I need: _____
_____

2. Tests to order: _____

_____

Progesterone
When to Use/How much to use? _____ What kind? _____

Estrogen prescription
When to Use/How much to use? _____ What kind? _____

Testosterone prescription
When to Use/How much to use? _____ What kind? _____

Step Two: Discover Your Emotional Type

Read pages: 101–112

Which type are you?

❏ Revved up and Anxious Type

❏ I Can't Get off the Couch Type

❏ Combination Type

My Emotional Type is: _____

Nutritional support suggested for your type:

PLEASE NOTE: Take these supplements in addition to Mia's Basic Supplement Program (see next page).

Type of Supplement	Dose	When/How Often

Step Three: Food and Supplements to the Rescue

Read pages: 113–135

Mia's Basic Supplement Program

Everyone, regardless of their hormonal phase or emotional type, should take the following supplements. All other recommendations are intended as additional support to this basic program.

Nutritional Supplement	Dosage
Multivitamin	For recommended content see Step Three: Food and Supplements to the Rescue

The following recommendations are the daily total amounts including what you might get in your multivitamin.

Vitamin B_{12}	1000–2000 mcg
Folic Acid	800 mcg
Vitamin B_6	50–100 mg
EPA Omega-3	600 mg
DHA Omega-3	400 mg
Calcium	500–800 mg
Magnesium Chelate	400–600 mg
Vitamin D_3	2000–3000 IU
Probiotics See Step Three: Food and Supplements to the Rescue for specific recommendations	10–20 billion organisms

Foods to Enjoy (see pages 128–132): _____

_____

_____

_____

_____

Foods to Avoid (see pages 132–135): _____

_____

_____

_____

_____

Step Four: Stress-buster and Life-improvement Techniques

Read pages: 137–155

Make a list of your top five stressors in your life (read page 138).

My Five Top Stressors:

1. _____

2. _____

3. _____

4. _____

5. _____

Change the Way Your Body Responds to Stress

Choose one or two of the following healing modalities and schedule an appointment with an appropriate health care practitioner (read pages 139–142).

___ Biofeedback

___ Neurolinguistic Programming (NLP)

___ Acupuncture

___ Hypnosis

Practice the following antidotes to stress. Some of the remedies you can incorporate into your daily life, others you might want to do on a weekly schedule. Circle a few remedies that you are willing to try.

- Take time to breathe
- Love yourself and others
- Hug a lot
- Stroke a pet
- Laugh
- Pray
- Get counseling
- Listen to a meditation CD
- Take a yoga class
- Try art or music therapy
- Join a community (church, spiritual organizations, parent groups, support groups)
- Lower the bar; stop being a perfectionist
- Sleep more
- Take naps
- Walk in nature
- Cultivate new friends and nurture old ones
- Take some time for yourself today, even one minute
- Do less
- Get a massage
- Take a bath

What are your three wishes for contentment? (Read page 151).

1. _____

2. _____

3. _____

Create your own "honey-do" list (read pages 152–153).

- _____
- _____
- _____

*** Optional Steps Five and Six ***

Steps Five and Six require you to take some diagnostic tests to determine your need for adrenal or thyroid support.

Step Five: Adrenal Health

- Read pages: 159–181.
- Send away for a simple lab kit and determine if you need adrenal support.
- Order you own saliva test to do at home or ask your doctor to order it. (Read pages 177–178 for testing information.)

My Adrenal Test Results:

Cortisol: _____ (high or low)

DHEA-S: _____ (high or low)

Nutritional Supplements for Adrenal Support

Make sure you follow the recommendations based on your test results (pages 179–181).

Type of Supplement	Dose	When

Step Six: Thyroid Support

Read pages: 183–196.

Ask your doctor for a thyroid blood test panel. Guidelines and reference values for test results found on pages 192.

My thyroid test results:

THS: Normal/high/low (circle what applies)

Free T4: Normal/high/low (circle what applies)

Free T3: Normal/high/low (circle what applies)

Reverse T3: Normal/high/low (circle what applies)

Thyroid Peroxidase Antibodies (TPO): Normal/high (circle what applies)

Anti-thyroid Antibodies: Normal/high (circle what applies)

• Fill in the following chart if your doctor gives you a prescription for thyroid hormone replacement.

Thyroid Hormone Replacement Prescribed by My Doctor

Type of Thyroid Hormone Replacement	Dose	When

Foods to avoid that could block thyroid function (read page 193):

• _____

• _____

• _____

Foods to incorporate in my diet that might support thyroid function (read page 193):

• _____

• _____

• _____

Good job! You now have completed your Emotional Rescue Plan. It won't take long to feel back in balance again.

Notes: _____

_____

_____

_____

_____

_____

_____

_____

Purchase What You Need

• With your Emotional Rescue Plan in hand, you can either go to your local health food store or shop online at www.femalebraingone insane.com for the food and supplements you need to get back to sanity (see Step Three).

Before you run off to the store, let me assure you that within the next few weeks you will have fewer symptoms and will start feeling much better. After you experience relief, please read the Afterword: Staying Sane—How to Maintain Emotional Balance for Life for a life-long maintenance plan.

Your needs will change as you move through life. If you stop and take time to pay attention to your symptoms, they will tell you when you need help and support. Your symptoms indicate specific needs and deficiencies. So never get so busy that you forget to listen to your body.

Mia's Mantras

Before you do anything else, read and practice Mia's Mantras. Repeat the following positive messages to yourself throughout the day. You deserve constant reassurance. Look for them throughout the book and believe.

- You will get better.
- You are not going crazy.
- It is just your chemistry.
- You are safe.
- You are not going off the deep end.
- You are a wonderful human being.
- You are strong.
- You have the power to change.

Part One

The Science Behind the Insanity and the Solution

Why the Female Brain Goes Insane

RIGHT NOW, I SUSPECT YOU FEEL emotionally out of balance. You might snicker, "That's an understatement." I'm sure you want to take immediate action to get back on track with your life, but it's important you recognize that a huge part of getting well is to understand what is going on beyond your unpleasant symptoms. Education is a powerful tool when it comes to healing. After many of my patients' initial consultations, they tell me "I feel better already," as they walk out the door. Why? Because learning why you feel the way you do will affect how you view your condition. No longer burdened by the worry of going insane, you can take charge and move forward. It's a good feeling to embrace something you haven't felt in so long—hope.

This chapter is designed to give you a dose of hope as you learn about how your female hormones change your brain chemistry and how the changes in your brain chemistry determine your emotional state or mood. It will answer many questions and provide solid solutions as well. How does the brain work? What are the brain chemicals that, when out of balance, create all of those emotional symptoms that make you feel like you're losing it? How does estrogen affect brain chemistry? How and why do you lose your emotional balance, and what can you do about it?

Meet Rebecca

"I was always a confident and zesty woman. Life was interesting, and I was busy and involved. But slowly, over many months, I found myself feeling flat and dull. I couldn't make a single decision. I'd wake up at 5 AM absolutely dreading the day. I'd mask the way I felt with a double latte, but within a few hours, I'd crave more coffee, garlic, and stimulation—anything to make me feel alive. I'd take walks and cry until my eyes turned inside out. What was going on? Yes, I had suffered the end of a meaningful relationship. Yes, a parent had died. I was grieving, but my anxious brooding was excessive, and I found no peace. Nothing could snap me out of this painful funk. I assumed my response to life's changes was normal, but my typical resilience, humor, and philosophic bent had completely disappeared. Who was I? I felt like a fragile shell of my former self, a disconnected, dark, negative woman. I was terrified. Was I falling apart?

"The days seemed to go on forever and I couldn't wait to lie down at night so that I could simply disappear. I considered having a blood test for my female hormones but my menopausal symptoms—nasty night sweats and very dry eyes—had stopped bothering me, so I assumed I was done and didn't need to wear my estrogen patch anymore. Alone and depressed, I figured I was another one of those middle-aged casualties, a woman in her mid-fifties who was going insane.

"I went to a psychiatrist who told me I was clinically depressed. He treated me with Zoloft, an SSRI. I was terribly agitated by the drug, but was convinced if I just took a little more I'd be fine. Even though the dose was raised from 50 to 400 milligrams, I found no relief. Instead I lost my appetite, wept, and fretted all day long.

"It was a long nightmare with no end until I finally found Mia. She listened to my symptoms and my story of sadness and depression and told me she understood! She assured me I was not alone! Then she ran some tests and discovered I had absolutely no estrogen and my neurotransmitters serotonin and dopamine, responsible for feelings of well-being and happiness, were depleted as well.

"I was immediately put on a dose of estrogen (I began with injections and gradually weaned off and used topical gels) and within only a couple of days stopped weeping and began to feel some ground under my feet. I titrated off the Zoloft and began taking an amino acid called 5-HTP to give my body the building blocks it needed to make serotonin. Two weeks later I added another amino acid called tyrosine to increase my neurotransmitter dopamine. I began eating protein in the morning and doing some biofeedback work. Within a month I became stable, woke up without panic, and even started to laugh again. What a relief to feed my body what it needed and to come back to life!"

You Deserve to Be Heard

In 1900 BC Egypt, a condition attributed to "the wandering of the uterus," was recorded by ancient physicians on stone slabs. It was called hysteria, from the Greek word for womb. Over time, that definition has grown to encompass any uncontrollable outburst of emotion or fear, often characterized by irrationality or excessive weeping. It became a catchall term for female mental disorders, and in the Middle Ages, it was associated with witchcraft and demonic possessions. In early psychiatry, the "irrational" behavior of a woman was reason enough for a hysterectomy, even if there were no physical problems or pathology present. Unbelievable though it may seem, in the twenty-first century, women around the world are still institutionalized for what we now know as a neuroendocrine (neuro meaning brain and endocrine meaning hormone) imbalance. Now, we hear negative words and phrases such as hormonal, irrational, or out of control to describe this imbalance.

Emotional symptoms due to hormonal and brain chemistry imbalances can mirror certain psychiatric illnesses. Naturally some women need serious psychiatric therapy and medication. However, I believe many traditional health care practitioners do not listen to women's symptoms and will offer medications to quiet them down instead of addressing the root cause of the distress. I believe this approach is unacceptable and does not work. *Female Brain Gone Insane,* on the other hand, offers a proven solution to better health.

Depression, anxiety, and mood swings can be devastating in all areas of a woman's life. Emotional imbalance affects your family, relationships, career, and your ability to have fun and just plain relax. Many women still believe their symptoms are not real, and they try to ignore them or shake them off. These inaccurate beliefs can discourage some women with depression and other true disorders from seeking treatment. Having emotional issues is not a sign of personal weakness or lack of character. You feel the way you do because of a biochemical imbalance in your brain. When a woman has diabetes or low thyroid she'll seek treatment and take insulin or thyroid hormones without guilt, but when it comes to depression or anxiety, some women feel ashamed of their condition. It's time to stop feeling lost or ashamed and address one of the key reasons you just don't feel right—your brain chemistry is out of balance.

Psychologists and neurobiologists frequently debate whether negative thinking, stressful events (abuse, dysfunctional family, etc.), or biological processes cause depression and anxiety. I believe the mind, however, does not exist without the brain. Considerable evidence indicates that regardless of the initial triggers, the final common pathway to feeling out of sorts involves biochemical changes in the brain. In other words, the changes in your brain chemistry make you feel the way you do. Stressors of any type can trigger your body's nervous system into a stress response. No matter the cause, your nervous system will respond the same to long-term stress. Your adrenal glands will release the stress hormones cortisol and adrenaline, and your serotonin levels eventually drop. These biochemical changes cause how you feel.

I know you may feel as if you have lost control over your own emotions, like the rug has been pulled out from underneath your trembling legs. But when you understand that these feelings are the result of too little or too much of a brain chemical, I hope you can breathe a sigh of relief. Yes, there is something tangible going on. Yes, there is a real reason you feel anxious or sad, and yes, there are brain-mood foods, supplements, and hormones that can make a real change in how you feel. There is a solution. When you feel anxious and out of sorts, you need to hear this one hundred times a day!

Mia's Mantra
You **will** get better

Your Nervous System

Your nervous system is complex. It consists of the central nervous system—your brain and spinal cord—and the peripheral nervous system, which runs throughout the rest of your body. Your brain contains billions of nerve cells arranged in patterns that coordinate thought, emotion, behavior, movement, and sensation. This complicated highway system of nerves helps your brain communicate with the rest of your body.

Your peripheral nervous system consists of all the other nerves in your body and links the brain to the organs, tissues, and glands through the spinal cord. The peripheral nervous system is a communication relay between your brain and your extremities. If you touch a hot stove, for example, signals travel from your finger to your brain in a split second and your brain instantly tells the muscles in your arm, *ouch, that's hot* and instructs your hand to remove your finger right away! In another example, when you sense danger the brain communicates with the peripheral system to mobilize the rest of your body to get ready to fight or flight. Muscles tense, palms sweat, the heart beats quicker, and you breathe faster as your body reacts by fighting or running.

Neurotransmitters

Neurotransmitters are naturally occurring chemical messengers that transmit information from one nerve cell to another, allowing the brain cells to talk to one another. Neurotransmitters control your behavior, so an imbalance or lack of certain neurotransmitters makes you feel lousy and out of sorts. Brain chemicals used to be a mystery, but today we can measure the levels of brain chemicals and manipulate them with natural supplements.

For the intricate and complex web of the nervous system to function and communicate properly, impulses have to travel rapidly from one cell to another. But nerve cells are not completely attached to one another. There are tiny little gaps between each cell called synapses. The nerve cell right before the space or synapse is called a presynaptic cell. The vesicles on this cell release the neurotransmitter. The nerve cell adjacent to the synapse is called the postsynaptic cell. The receptors on this cell receive the neurotransmitter. This process is repeated from nerve cell to nerve cell, as an impulse travels to its destination. This amazing system makes it possible to move, think, feel, and communicate; it is also enables the heart to beat, the lungs to breathe, the intestines to digest, and certain glands to produce hormones.

Inhibitory neurotransmitters act like a brake pedal in your body and are generally responsible for calming the mind and body, inducing sleep, and filtering out unnecessary excitatory signals. Excitatory neurotransmitters act like an accelerator in your body and are responsible for providing energy, motivation, mental cognition, and other activities that require brain-body activity. A balance between the stimulating (excitatory) neurotransmitters and the calming (inhibitory) neurotransmitters is necessary for optimal health.

There are over fifty different neurotransmitters present in the nervous system, but only a handful are both measurable and understood to a degree that is relevant and applicable to personal health. These include serotonin, gamma-aminobutyric acid (GABA), norepinephrine, dopamine, epinephrine, histamine, agmatine, glutamate, phenylethylamine, glycine, aspartate, acetylcholine, and nitric oxide. Four of these neurotransmitters play a huge part in determining your mental and physical health and your sense of well-being. They are the inhibitory neurotransmitters serotonin and GABA, and the excitatory neurotransmitters norepinephrine and dopamine.

It is critical that there are enough of the major neurotransmitters present daily in order for the brain to be chemically balanced and for you to feel right emotionally. It is equally important that the inhibitory and excitatory neurotransmitters be in balance.

Neurotransmitters can change depending on your body's current requirements and circumstances. At night, the brain needs to raise the levels of the calming neurotransmitters to relax you so you can fall asleep. In the morning, it must lower the levels of these neurotransmitters and raise the levels of the excitatory neurotransmitters so you can focus and get going. Sleep disorders and lack of motivation indicate brain chemistry imbalances.

Some of the most significant clinical issues (and symptoms) linked to an imbalance of the excitatory and inhibitory neurotransmitters are:

- Anxiousness
- Appetite control
- Attention issues
- Behavioral problems
- Depression
- Fatigue
- Hormonal changes
- Headaches
- Libido
- Mood disorders
- Sleep disorders
- Weight control

Inhibitory Neurotransmitters

Serotonin is a key chemical that contributes to feelings of well-being and happiness. It also helps defend your system against both anxiety and depression. The level of serotonin in your body defines how you feel in many significant ways.

With normal levels of serotonin you may feel:

• Happy
• A sense of well-being
• Mellow and relaxed
• Hopeful and optimistic
• At peace
• Creative and thoughtful
• Solid impulse control; can say "no" more easily
• Reduced sensitivity to pain
• Deep restful sleep
• Secure and safe

With low levels of serotonin you may feel:

• Angry, irritable, filled with rage
• Violent and antisocial behavior
• Can't sleep well, insomnia
• Anxious
• Panicky
• Rapid thoughts
• Decreased interest in sex
• Carbohydrate and sugar cravings
• Alcohol cravings
• Headaches and migraines
• Aches and pains
• Intestinal distress

Some experts believe that low serotonin has become a virtual epidemic in the United States. Serotonin is the key to our feelings of happiness, and it helps defend against both anxiety and depression. That said, it is no surprise that a serotonin imbalance is one of the most common contributors to mood problems. When you have too little, you will usually feel uneasy, distressed, and highly emotional or agitated. Often, depression can occur in women because of low serotonin in combination with fluctuating estrogen levels, which may explain why some women have increased emotional imbalances during postpartum, premenstrual, and menopausal times.

In the central nervous system, serotonin acts as a calming neurotransmitter, and one of its main roles is to balance and control the other stimulating neurotransmitters. Together with the neurotransmitter GABA it prevents over-excitation. It also plays an important role in the inhibition of anger, aggression, and body-temperature fluctuations, as well as affecting mood, sleep patterns, sexuality, and appetite. Serotonin is also active in the peripheral nervous system.

Ninety-five percent of the body's serotonin is actually housed in the stomach and the intestines (gut)! It is no wonder Dr. Michael Gershon, chairman of the department of anatomy and cell biology at Columbia University, refers to the gut as "the second brain." Epithelial cells that line the gut secrete serotonin where it acts as a neurotransmitter and a signaling mechanism. It makes sense that many patients with anxiety and depression experience gastrointestinal tract discomfort. Serotonin is known to play an important role in irritable bowel syndrome (IBS), one of the most debilitating gastrointestinal disorders, characterized by cramping and bloating in some patients, or alternating diarrhea and constipation in others.

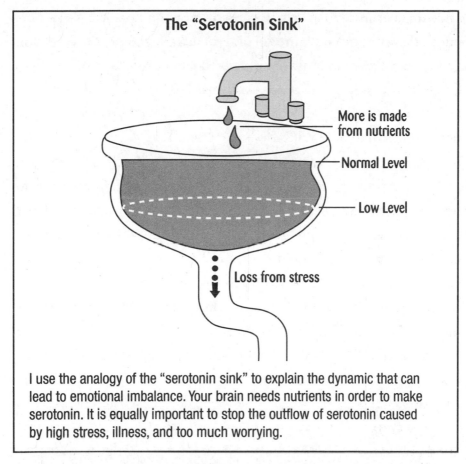

The "Serotonin Sink"

More is made
from nutrients

Normal Level

Low Level

Loss from stress

I use the analogy of the "serotonin sink" to explain the dynamic that can lead to emotional imbalance. Your brain needs nutrients in order to make serotonin. It is equally important to stop the outflow of serotonin caused by high stress, illness, and too much worrying.

Primarily a calming neurotransmitter in the brain, GABA is considered the body's natural tranquilizer. Rather than encouraging communication between cells as dopamine, serotonin, or norepinephrine do, GABA reduces, discourages, and blocks communication. GABA calms the brain by inhibiting over-excitement and helps induce relaxation and sleep and reduced anxiety. Low levels of GABA can occur because of prolonged GABA depletion, usually after long-term stress. Too little GABA in the brain causes chaotic communication between cells, resulting in over stimulation, which leads to anxiety, rage, and insomnia.

Women with high levels of GABA are often stressed out and exhibit symptoms of insomnia, anxiety, nervousness, and panic attacks. The body releases more and more GABA as it attempts to calm itself down. Too much GABA can cause too much relaxation and sedation, often to the point that normal reactions are impaired.

Excitatory Neurotransmitters

The stimulating (excitatory) neurotransmitters are like the accelerator in your car. When the excitatory neurotransmitter system is in drive, your system gets revved up for action. These neurotransmitter levels also increase during times of stress and fear. Without a functioning inhibitory system to put on the brakes (too little serotonin and GABA), the stimulating neurotransmitters take off and you can fly out of control, spinning into nervousness and anxiety. The key excitatory neurotransmitters are dopamine and norepinephrine.

The level of dopamine in your body defines how you feel in many significant ways. With high levels of dopamine you may feel:

• Anxiety
• Fear
• Feeling of detachment
• Sleep disturbances
• Panic attacks
• Increased sex drive
• Paranoia
• High blood pressure

With low levels of dopamine you may feel:

• Fatigue, low energy
• Depression, deep sadness
• The need for more sleep
• Withdrawn

- Difficulty focusing and concentrating
- Poor memory
- Suicidal or preoccupation with thoughts of suicide

The brain uses dopamine to create a heightened state of alertness, awareness, and aggression, and it is responsible for motivation, interest, and drive. When dopamine is elevated we think, speak, and breathe more rapidly. Dopamine is also associated with positive stress states, such as being in love, exercising, listening to music, and sex. When we don't have enough of it we feel dull and disinterested; we have difficulty initiating or completing tasks, experience poor concentration, and also lose energy and motivation. Dopamine doesn't just stimulate the brain, it is also is involved in muscle control and function. Low dopamine levels can prompt you to self medicate with drugs, alcohol, cigarettes, gambling, or food. On the other hand, high dopamine levels can lead to poor gastrointestinal function, mood swings, psychosis, and attention disorders in children.

Estrogen, tyrosine (amino acid), certain foods (protein rich foods such as meats, milk products, fish, beans, nuts, soy products), vigorous aerobic exercise, thoughts and images of excitement, risk-taking, gambling, and sexual arousal can increase dopamine levels.

Norepinephrine, also known as noradrenalin, is an excitatory neurotransmitter that becomes elevated during stress. It is most active when we are awake and contributes to our focused attention and good memory. The release of too much norepinephrine causes the sensations of nervousness, fluttery chest, palpitations, and sweating, which feel like the typical fight-or-flight stress response. The brain becomes stimulated, and women report feeling as if they can't stop thinking or can't turn off their brain. If these symptoms occur in the absence of a stressful situation, it can be frightening, especially when they occur in the middle of the night and interrupt sleep.

With high levels of norepinephrine you may feel:

• Stressed out
• Anxious
• High blood pressure
• Aggressive
• Manic

With low levels of norepinephrine you may feel:

• Depressed
• Apathetic
• Unfocused
• Lack of energy
• Lack of motivation
• Poor memory

The Causes of Brain Chemistry Imbalance

Medical research has shown that many factors associated with today's fast-paced lifestyle contribute to imbalances in neurotransmitter and hormone levels. Chronic stress serves as the primary contributor to neurotransmitter imbalance. Stress depletes certain neurotransmitters and increases the amounts of other neurotransmitters to help us cope with the many situations in our amped-up lives! It doesn't matter if the stress is from traffic, arguments, a high pressure job, a difficult relationship, a bacterial or viral infection, too much exercise, hormonal imbalances, or nutritional deficiency—all stressors are perceived the same by the nervous system. When your body identifies stress, it goes through a series of biochemical responses, which change the balance of the neurotransmitters. Acute stress is generally tolerated very well and doesn't cause significant neurotransmitter imbalances. But chronic stress creates a domino effect of serious biochemical changes leading to severe depression, complete adrenal burnout, and altered immune function.

Another common cause of neurotransmitter imbalance is hormone fluctuation and depletion. Estrogen, progesterone, and testosterone have a direct influence on both excitatory and inhibitory neurotransmitters. Estrogen is one of women's most potent antidepressants, which explains the importance of addressing hormonal imbalances in women who suffer emotionally. Poor dietary habits also contribute to neurotransmitter imbalances, especially when combined with high stress. The production of neurotransmitters depends on adequate levels of amino acid precursors. As an example, the amino acid tyrosine is needed make dopamine, and tryptophan to make serotonin. Diets low in protein may limit the supplies of these amino acids, decreasing neurotransmitter levels. If your nutrition is poor and you do not take in enough protein, vitamins, or minerals, you will not manufacture enough neurotransmitters.

Our brain cell membranes are composed primarily of lipids, which are also known as fats. Omega-3 fatty acids stabilize these membranes and are required for proper brain cell function. Diets low in these fatty acids can compromise the integrity of the neurons themselves and lead to faulty neurotransmission. We really are not just what we eat, but what we absorb. Faulty metabolism and digestive issues can impair absorption and breakdown of our food, which will reduce our ability to build neurotransmitters.

Neurological toxins are another major contributor to neurotransmitter imbalances. Toxic substances like heavy metals, industrial solvents, pesticides, drug and alcohol abuse, and some prescription drugs can cause permanent damage to the nerve cells that make neurotransmitters. Because some of these chemical toxins are lipid-soluble and the brain is composed mainly of lipids, many toxins find their way past the blood-brain barrier and into brain cells. Once a toxin reaches the brain cell, it can cause significant imbalances in brain chemistry.

The last major influence of neurotransmitter imbalances is genetic factors. Some individuals are metabolically predisposed to neurotransmitter deficiencies or excesses resulting in drug or alcohol abuse, eating disorders, attention deficit and hyperactivity disorders, or mood disorders that run in families. A combination of chronic stress, poor diet, neurotoxins, and genetics can create neurotransmitter-related conditions. When the cause of the neurotransmitter imbalance is stress or poor diet, addressing these issues can eliminate the need for neurotransmitter support. However, when the neurotransmitter imbalance is due to a genetic predisposition or a neuro-toxic exposure, the need for neurotransmitter support may be ongoing.

Regardless of the cause, you and your health care practitioner can now test your neurotransmitters levels to determine which ones are responsible for the brain chemistry imbalances causing your emotional distress. In addition, your emotional symptoms also clearly tell you what your brain chemistry wants and needs. Once you know which neurotransmitters are too high or too low, you can figure out the kind of support you need—from amino acids and other nutritional supplements and mood foods, to hormones and lifestyle changes—to help you stop feeling insane and begin to find your emotional balance again.

The Hormone and Brain Chemistry Dance

The root of your symptoms revolves around the dance between your female hormones and brain chemistry during hormonal shifts throughout your life. Your hormones and neurotransmitters, as chemical messengers, relay vital instructions throughout you entire body. Hormones are like the big-shot directors on a movie set telling the cells—who are like the actors with different important functions to act out—what they need to do. Each cell responds by playing her part in the making of a seamless, hopefully engaging Lifetime movie. As hormones travel throughout the body and brain, they direct the cells to work faster or slower to perform their particular functions. All of our hormones are designed to work as an ensemble, to perform in harmony with each other as well as with nature's circadian rhythms, night and day cycles, and seasons. When they do not execute their particular tasks or operate below par, things start to unravel and we can feel it.

There are many types of hormones, but our primary focus is on estrogen and progesterone—the two key female hormones that define your sense of wholeness, well-being, and health—and are secreted into the bloodstream at different times in a woman's cycle. Estrogen has a profound effect on the brain and the brain chemistry. In early perimenopause, women often experience erratic or high levels of estrogen. Usually we concern ourselves with the unpleasant symptoms of too little estrogen, but too much estrogen can contribute to feelings of rage, irritability, and anxiety. Progesterone can counteract these symptoms and contribute to a woman's sense of ease because it has a tranquilizing effect on mood by increasing GABA in the brain. Too much progesterone can cause feelings of tiredness and even sedation, but it can be used to help women who are feeling anxious and irritable.

As you can see, hormones do not operate in isolation. They are intricately involved with the neurotransmitters in our brain that tell us when to sleep, when to get focused, when to eat, when to slow down, and when to have sex. One does not dance without the other, and neither do we! Before we discuss how hormones can work together in perfect syn-copation or step on one another's toes, we need to take a brief peek at the profound synergy of estrogen and serotonin.

Estrogen and Serotonin: The Female Dynamic Duo

Estrogen is well known for building the curves that create a woman's shapely figure and for activating and overseeing the female reproductive system. But estrogen's role in female health goes far beyond reproduction. Almost all women can recall a few dramatic stories of how they felt out-of-character while premenstrual (one to two weeks before the period starts), when estrogen levels drop and the hormonal balance is sometimes thrown off. During the premen-strual weeks, some women go over the edge and feel terrible—well beyond the minor discomfort of feeling cranky, bloated, or irritable. In some cases, they experience upsetting panic attacks, bulimics binge and purge more frequently, kleptomaniacs engage in more stealing escapades, hair pullers pull more hair out, skin cutters cut more skin.

All of these behaviors are related to a dramatic drop in estrogen, which causes a deficiency of the neurotransmitter serotonin, the feel-good chemical. When a woman makes enough serotonin she feels content, happy, and at peace. Serotonin and estrogen are a dynamic duo, functioning in tandem. As your estrogen levels drop, so do sero-tonin levels, and you may feel agitated, anxious, and irritable. When estrogen levels start to rise (as they do during the second week of the menstrual cycle) the amount of serotonin available in the spaces between the brain's nerve cells increases. This improves mood and restoring calm. A normal and stable level of estrogen is needed for serotonin function and production, while enough serotonin allows for adequate estrogen production by the ovaries.

Serving as a brain booster, a natural antidepressant, and mood stabilizer, estrogen affects all levels of serotonin functioning. For example:

- Estrogen makes tryptophan (one of the building blocks of serotonin) more available in the brain to create serotonin.
- Estrogen increases the destruction of the enzyme monoamine oxidase (MAO). The lower your MAO enzyme levels, the better you probably feel, since MAO breaks down serotonin so you can not use it in your brain.
- Estrogen increases the retrieval of serotonin by increasing the efficiency of serotonin receptors.

Hadine Joffe, M.D., and Lee Cohen, M.D., two researchers in the Perinatal and Reproductive Psychiatry Program at Harvard Medical School, conducted over one hundred studies on the relationship between women's hormonal cycles and their mental status to determine the connection between female hormones and brain chemistry health. In study after study, they confirmed that women with histories of depression were apparently more vulnerable to recurrent episodes during periods of what the researchers call "significant reproductive endocrine change," meaning after childbirth, premenstrually, during perimenopause, and menopause, when estrogen drops are most significant.

Another important study published in the *American Journal of Psychiatry* showed that 41 percent of the women admitted into an inpatient psychiatric hospital checked in the day before or the first day of menses, when estrogen levels are at their lowest.

In order to maintain balance, harmony, and well-being a woman needs the right combination of bioidentical hormones at the right time of her menstrual cycle. She also needs the right kind and amount of nutritional supplements (including amino acid therapy) to rebalance levels of the neurotransmitters serotonin, GABA, dopamine, and norepinephrine. Health care practitioners treating women with emotional symptoms need to be aware that the synergy of hormones and brain chemistry support is the key to creating emotional well-being.

Now that you have a better understanding of why you feel the way you do, you can begin to feel hopeful about the positive results you'll get from designing and using Your Emotional Rescue Plan.

2

The Bioidentical Hormone Solution

THIS CHAPTER TEACHES YOU ABOUT bioidentical hormones so that you understand what they really are, how they affect your brain, and why they are safe. Although bioidentical hormones have recently become popular, I have prescribed them for almost twenty years along with nutritional therapies and lifestyle changes. During that time, I am proud to have helped thousands of women rebalance their bodies and brains with great success.

As you enter your mid-thirties to fifties, you produce less estrogen, progesterone, and testosterone. Women's ovaries are programmed to shrivel up—though not an appealing image, the ovaries do go from looking like flower blossoms to raisins. Sorry. It's the truth. So, for most of you, by fifty years old, halfway through a potentially long life, you find yourself without enough of the female hormones needed to remain healthy and vibrant. As a result, many systems in your body work with less efficiency.

For example, as blood flow to your brain lessens your brain function declines. You may feel as if you live inside of a Jell-O mold—some call it brain fog—often typified by occasionally forgetting the names of people and things you've known your entire life. The little blood vessels called coronary arteries that feed your heart with blood may begin to clog, leading to angina and heart attacks. The juices in your gut that promote the absorption of nutrients diminish and you may experience symptoms such as bloating or flatulence. Your skin and vaginal tissue may begin dry, and your joints may get squeaky. Sound familiar?

Based on recent research and years of clinical practice, I have no doubt that the right balance of bioidentical hormones keeps your brain focused, your body in better health, and your soul happy. With bioidentical hormones you can lower the risk of age-related disease: your cholesterol levels and the development of coronary artery plaque will remain low, resulting in a significant decrease in the likelihood of developing cardiovascular disease. The lining in your intestines will stay healthy, which can prevent irritable bowel problems and other intestinal disorders, such as colon cancer. Bioidentical hormones also prevent your hair from falling out, your bones from becoming brittle, your joints from drying out, and your waist from going bye-bye. It's pretty amazing, and a true blessing to have access to these hormones. By replacing the hormones that you lack with bioidentical hormones, I am certain you will enjoy a healthier second half of life.

Many books and current health fads promote radical hormone replacement therapy with what I consider unrealistic and almost ridiculous promises. The proponents believe more is better. Their premise is: why not rev up the hormones of a woman in her fifties to mimic that of a typical healthy twenty-five-year-old? I take issue with this approach. My basic philosophy is: replace the hormones to a level where the body is humming along again, without symptoms and without side effects that can result from levels that are too high. More is not necessarily better. *The goal is always balance.*

I find most patients in my practice experience relief and feel as well as they used to feel or better by replacing the estrogen to an estradiol serum levels of 50 to 150 pg/mL (some patients might need a little more for normal brain and body function).

About 150 years ago (a blink of the eye in human history) life expectancy was only forty-seven to forty-eight years of age. Women would reproduce, take care of their offspring, and then die, often before menopause. Back then, a tooth infection could mean the end of life. Today with advances in hygiene, science, and medicine, we certainly hang on much longer and can actually expect to live, and live well, for another thirty to fifty years after menopause. Women's life expectancy is now eighty-one years of age.

With new knowledge about human physiology and stress, we now have the power to outsmart Mother Nature. It's time to take advantage of what we've learned and take charge. To do this, women can put back their natural hormones during those thirty to forty "unnatural" years of our new longer lives. We can slow down aging and degeneration, along with reducing the risk of osteoporosis, dementia, heart attacks, and colon cancer. At the same time we can feel vibrant again, and that means we can feel sexy, smart, and in control of our own emotions.

Drug Versus Bioidentical Hormone Replacement Therapy

Over the last decade, more and more women express concern about what hormones they need, if they are safe, and how long to take them. For so many years, doctors doled out synthetic hormones and horse estrogens as a matter of course. The truth is that the medical community has acted at times quite blindly. So much misleading information comes from pharmaceutically sponsored studies that have their own profit-promoting agenda in mind. Today, women are more educated about hormones and want natural ways to treat symptoms of hormonal imbalance.

I believe women need hormones that look and act as closely as possible to what their bodies naturally produce. That is, they need bioidentical hormones. Virtually all researchers agree that women should not hesitate to use hormone replacement therapy, commonly called HRT, to mitigate their symptoms when menopause begins. Many experts recommend the use of hormones to alleviate symptoms of PMS and perimenopause. Now, all doctors have access to human bioidentical hormones but many choose not to use them. Instead, doctors prescribe estrogens such as Premarin. As the name implies, *Pre-mar-in* is derived from the urine of pregnant mares. The mares are kept in tight quarters where their urine is collected through a catheter inserted in the horse's bladder. So the estrogens in Premarin are natural to horses, not to women! It's probably a great treatment for menopause if you have four hooves and a tail, but you don't.

Premarin is often prescribed in combination with the synthetic progesterone called Provera, This combination is actually drug replacement therapy, not hormone replacement therapy. Often women end up suffering from a myriad of side effects and receive no symptom relief. Most often, doctors offer no alternatives, and women are left in despair.

Bioidentical Hormones Demystified

Herbs and plants grow in nature and are natural in their own habitats. However, they are not a natural part of our bodies. By taking herbs such as red clover, black cohosh, and dong quai to alleviate symptoms of hormonal imbalance, you are not treating the cause, which is a lack of hormones.

During our reproductive years, our ovaries make estrogen, progesterone, and testosterone. The most natural hormone replacement therapy would be to extract and bottle up our own hormones during our reproductive years and inject them back into our bodies after menopause. In ancient China, the older women suffering from menopausal symptoms drank younger women's urine to alleviate symptoms. This actually worked because women in their reproductive years do excrete estrogens in their urine! Since we do not (yet) follow those practices in the Western world today, the closest we can get to applying, ingesting, or injecting what is natural to our human bodies, is through bioidentical hormones. The molecules of the bioidentical hormone look identical to the molecules of the hormones our ovaries used to make in great quantity.

Interestingly, bioidentical hormones are made in the laboratory. Yes, they are derived from plant sources, meaning the plant hormone is extracted from the plant and then synthesized or tweaked in lab to look exactly like the hormones made by your ovaries. Analogously, these hormones are the right key for the right lock. Your body says, "Hello. I recognize you." Then the bioidentical hormone key finds the receptor, unlocks it, and voila! Once the hormones are in place, your body can stop screaming for what it needs and can shift back into balance. You feel good again. To hit home the point: Bioidentical hormone replacement therapy essentially puts back hormones that perfectly fit into our cell receptors, and the body welcomes them back as if they were our own. Hormones do not have to be compounded by a compounding pharmacy to be bioidentical. Bioidentical hormones are also commercially made. (See Step One: Identify Your Hormonal

Phase for specifics.) However, compounding pharmacies can formulate specific dosages that might not be available commercially.

Synthetic hormones are manmade and do not resemble anything from nature. They are not hormones, they are drugs. Since drug companies cannot patent bioidentical hormones, they add synthetic molecules to bioidentical hormones to create an end product that looks different from nature and can therefore be patented. However, your body knows it isn't the real deal. It is a sorry state of affairs because bioidentical hormones are readily available for doctors by prescription, at any regular or compounding pharmacy, yet doctors continue to prescribe women estrogen derived from horse urine and synthetic progesterone.

Make no mistake, birth control pills are not bioidentical hormones. They contain a very potent mixture of synthetic estrogen and synthetic progesterone that actually suppress your natural hormones, the very hormones that you need for emotional balance. In addition, the synthetic progesterone in birth control pills can cause a set of emotional symptoms such as agitation, irritability, and rage.

Estradiol

During a woman's reproductive life, her ovaries secrete three different estrogens: estrone, estradiol, and estriol. A substantial volume of scientific research clearly demonstrates estradiol is the key estrogen essential for optimal brain function. A brain booster, natural antidepressant, and mood stabilizer, estradiol supports healthy serotonin levels; and serotonin helps you sleep better, and feel calmer and happier. In addition, estradiol seems to protect brain cells from stress, injury, and damage implicated in the development of Alzheimer's disease. It also increases blood flow through the brain, which improves brain function, and it acts as an anti-inflammatory agent protecting blood vessel walls from plaque formation.

Progesterone

Progesterone is the first hormone that declines as we age. In our mid-to-late thirties, progesterone levels start to drop with the decline in ovulation. Low progesterone levels cause PMS and perimenopausal symptoms. While progesterone doesn't seem as crucial as estrogen when it comes to brain function, it does have a tranquilizing effect on mood because it increases the feel-calm neurotransmitter GABA in the brain. Research indicates that the brain makes fewer receptors for GABA during the time when progesterone is low in the menstrual cycle. This explains why women suffering from PMS often experience irritability, agitation, and anxiety. Since progesterone calms the nervous system, too much progesterone can cause lethargy or even mild depression.

Progesterone also keeps estrogen receptors functioning by making sure the receptors, like little keyholes, are ready to receive the estrogen keys. Without the progesterone, the little keyholes get "rusty." In some studies, progesterone was found to be the basic hormone that allows the body to adapt to and handle stress with more ease. In addition, progesterone prevents excessive production of the potentially harmful adrenal hormone cortisol, which, in chronically high levels, may lead to a plethora of other potential problems such as osteoporosis, aging of the skin, damage to brain cells, and the accumulation of fat around the waist and the back. That is why progesterone is often called the guardian hormone. Several studies indicate that bioidentical progesterone is protective when it comes to breast cancer. A recent French study indicates that by using bioidentical progesterone in combination with estrogen (in this study women had used a variety of estrogens, bioidentical, and Premarin), the possible increased risk of breast cancer was eliminated, indicating no increased risk of breast cancer compared to women who never had used estrogen.

Testosterone

Testosterone, known as the hormone of passion, can provide what estrogen alone cannot—renewed sexual desire. Both the ovaries and the adrenal glands produce it. When balanced correctly with estrogen, testosterone plays a lead role in making you feel good. Declining levels of testosterone play a direct role in decreased sexual desire and "flatness" of mood sometimes experienced during and after menopause. Testosterone not only boosts libido and energy, it also maintains muscle mass, strengthens bone, and makes sure the nipples and clitoris are sensitive to sexual pleasure. By age forty, women produce about half the testosterone that they did in their twenties. Testosterone levels drop further with the onset of menopause or when a woman's ovaries are removed.

Several studies suggest that small amounts of testosterone (taken orally or topically) used with estrogen replacement therapy can restore sexual desire, improve energy, promote a sense of well-being, and support cognitive function. Testosterone has a beneficial affect on the feel-good brain chemical dopamine, which increases your zest for life. It is also associated with positive stress states, such as being in love, exercising, listening to music, and having sex.

Is Hormone Replacement Safe?

Many women want to avoid taking HRT at all costs. They worry excessively about developing breast cancer. If you have these concerns, your anxiety may be misplaced. Your risk of having breast cancer is far lower than your risk of having or dying from cardiovascular disease. Heart disease is responsible for more deaths in women than all forms of cancer combined and is the most significant health concern for women in the United States today, causing nearly 350,000 deaths each year compared to only 40,000 from breast cancer.

What is even more concerning is that the media and many practitioners fail to tell you that certain hormones will reduce the risk of cardiovascular disease by as much as 60 percent without increasing your risk of breast cancer! This is good news. Sadly, the media focuses on reports of breast cancer run rampant without educating and warning women about the more imminent danger of heart disease.

Comparing Bioidentical to Synthetic Hormones

The media warns women about the risks of HRT *regardless of the type of hormones that were used in the studies.* No matter what type of hormones were used, bioidentical, synthetic, horse-derived hormones, oral or transdermal, when presented to you the consumer, they all fall under the umbrella of HRT, which gives every type of hormone replacement a bad name.

In 1994, the National Institute of Health began the Women's Health Initiative (WHI) study. The goal of the study was to evaluate the long-term effect of hormone replacement therapy versus placebo (sugar pill) in the prevention of heart disease, osteoporosis, breast cancer, and stroke in postmenopausal women. The only hormones used in the study were the horse estrogen Premarin and the synthetic progesterone Provera. Unfortunately, the WHI did not include a bioidentical hormone in the study. The WHI study came to an abrupt halt in July 2002 because the combination of the drugs Premarin and Provera also marketed as PremPro showed an increased risk of breast cancer, coronary heart disease, and stroke. Specifically, the study showed women who took these drugs had a 24 percent increased risk of breast cancer and an overall 24 percent increased risk of coronary heart disease then those who didn't.

What the media and most doctors fail to tell you is that the group of women in the study who took Premarin without Provera had no increased risk of breast cancer. In addition, after five years, the same group of women showed 61 percent less calcified plaque of their coronary arteries compared to the women who took a placebo. So according to the WHI study, taking Premarin without adding Provera was more beneficial when it came to heart disease and breast cancer than not taking any hormones at all!

Again, the WHI study clearly proved that synthetic progesterone, used in most HRT, causes breast cancer and heart disease. This was not news to me. A long history of studies show that synthetic progesterone like Provera will increase the risk of breast cancer while bioidentical progesterone will have a powerful protective effect against breast cancer. For this reason, I have been preaching the dangers of synthetic progesterone such as Provera for the last twenty years, while exclusively using bioidentical progesterone in my practice. Not one published scientific study indicates that bioidentical progesterone increases the risk of breast cancer. In fact, it is shown to have anticancer effects. However, synthetic progestins are known carcinogens.

Large-scale studies conducted in Europe on bioidentical hormones therapies repeatedly have demonstrated that bioidentical hormones effectively eliminate menopausal symptoms with a lack of long-term negative side effects. A large French study investigated the breast cancer risk factors in 1998 and found that bioidentical progesterone compared to synthetic progesterone was associated with significantly lower risks of breast cancer. Another French study on 3,175 postmenopausal women using mainly transdermal bioidentical estrogen and progesterone found that after 8.9 years the women had no increased risk of breast cancer.

One study published in the *Journal of the National Cancer Institute* found a lower risk of recurrence of breast cancer and deaths in women who used hormone replacement therapy after breast cancer diagnosis than women who did not, suggesting that HRT (unfortunately, again the researchers studied women who took either bioidentical or synthetic hormones without any differentiation) after breast cancer had no adverse impact on recurrence and mortality.

It is also clear from numerous studies that taking synthetic progesterone such as Provera will increase a women's risk of heart disease by blocking the protective effects of estrogen. On the other hand, bioidentical progesterone will add to the positive benefits of estrogen.

Premarin, when taken by mouth, travels through the liver and significantly increases the risk of blood clots, which can cause strokes and heart attacks. This risk is amplified when Provera is added. When estrogen is taken through the skin by patch or cream, this problem is eliminated, and there is no increased risk of clotting.

The third leading cause of death among women is colorectal cancer. Several studies that did not differentiate the types of hormones used, including the Nurses' Health Study and the WHI, showed that women currently using estrogen replacement therapy or HRT have a significantly lower risk of colorectal cancer. A new finding, published in the January 2009 issue of *Cancer Epidemiology, Biomarkers and Prevention*, found a 17 percent reduced risk of colorectal cancer among women who had at one time used estrogen, a 25 percent reduced risk among women currently using estrogen, and a 26 percent reduced risk among those using estrogen for ten or more years. Another study by Dr. Paganini-Hill analyzed the medical records of 7,701 women aged 44 to 98 in a Southern California retirement community and found that the women who had used estrogen had a 33 percent lower risk of colon cancer than those who had never used it.

A World Health Organization summary of studies regarding osteoporosis and hip fracture concluded that women who take estrogen for more than seven to ten years have a 50 percent lower risk of hip or wrist fracture and a 75 percent lower risk of vertebral fracture.

Kent Holtorf, M.D., wrote a very well researched paper published in *Post Graduate Medicine,* January 2009, where he reviewed numerous papers comparing the effects of bioidentical and the synthetic hormones. His conclusion was:

> A thorough review of the medical literature supports the claim that bioidentical hormones have some distinctly different, often opposite, physiological effects to those of their synthetic counterparts. With respect to the risk for breast cancer, heart disease, heart attack, and stroke, substantial scientific and medical evidence demonstrates that bioidentical hormones are safer and more efficacious forms of HRT than commonly used synthetic versions. More randomized control trials of substantial size and length will be needed to further delineate these differences.

As you can see, significant evidence exists in support of bioidentical hormones. Yet, the Food and Drug Administration represents there is little or no evidence to support claims that bioidentical hormones are safer than the synthetic hormones.

The First Global Summit on Menopause-related Issues, held in Zurich on March 29 and 30, 2008, involved forty of the world's leading menopause experts who met to review public perceptions, risks, and benefits of hormone replacement therapy (again, they did not distinguish between bioidentical and synthetic hormones). They looked at four main areas of controversy: cardiovascular health, breast issues, cognition, and bone issues. The Summit concluded HRT is safe and that healthy women going through the first few years of the menopause who need HRT to relieve symptoms should have no fears about its use.

The American Association of Clinical Endocrinologists and the North American Menopause Society have also come to similar conclusions. Further, Amos Pines, president of The International Menopause Society said in a 2007 press statement:

> Health-care providers should stay with the first-grade information coming from the WHI study when discussing this issue with their patients: breast-wise, in women younger than 60, [HRT] (particularly estrogen-alone) is safe [here again he is referring to Premarin without the synthetic progesterone Provera.] Long-term use may be associated with a small increased risk, in the order of one extra case per 1,000 women per year. Discontinuation of HT [he says HT meaning hormone therapy, same as HRT] brings this risk back to the values for age-matched non-users after three to five years. Weighing the overall benefits and risks of HT in the younger postmenopausal population clearly favors the use of HT for symptomatic women.

Unfortunately, many doctors seem unaware of the research in support of even Premarin estrogen replacement. They also misconstrued the results of the WHI believing women are better off not taking any hormone replacement therapy. Consequently, many women will need-lessly suffer from and be at increased risk for depression, heart disease, stroke, osteoporosis, and colon cancer.

Clearly, bioidentical hormones are very different from their synthetic versions, often having opposite (read: positive) physical and cellular effects, and that the bioidentical hormones do not pertain to the outcome of the WHI study. Based on what I have seen in my clinical practice in over 20 years of prescribing bioidentical hormones to my patients, bioidentical hormones—particularly the transdermal forms of estrogen—do not appear to have negative side effects or the risk profile associated with synthetic HRT. As much as I rely on my clinical experience, I always, always want to see the science to back it up. Clearly, more studies are needed.

Until there is evidence to the contrary, I believe bioidentical transdermal estradiol in combination with oral bioidentical progesterone should be the preferred method of HRT. In my practice, I have a few patients who cannot tolerate oral progesterone due to side effects such as sedation and depression. In these cases, I do prescribe transdermal or vaginal progesterone but require uterine cancer screening for the patients every six to twelve months.

Key Facts About Bioidentical Versus Synthetic HRT

- Synthetic progesterone such as Provera increases the risk of breast cancer and cardiovascular disease.
- One reason that Provera increases the risk of heart disease is that it is blocking the beneficial effects of estrogens (Premarin or bioidentical estrogen).

- In the WHI, women who took Premarin without Provera had a decreased incidence of breast cancer and cardiovascular disease compared to the women who took no hormones.
- Not one published study indicates that bioidentical progesterone increases the risk of breast cancer.
- Oral (taken by mouth) estrogen increases the risk of clotting and inflammation. This risk is amplified when taking Provera.
- When bioidentical estrogen is taken trough the skin, this risk is eliminated.
- The prospective, comparative Postmenopausal Estrogens/Progestin Intervention trial (PEPI study) has recommended oral bioidentical progesterone as the first choice for opposing estrogen therapy in post-menopausal women to prevent uterine cancer.
- Due to lack of substantial research on transdermal progesterone in the prevention of uterine cancer, oral bioidentical progesterone should be the recommended type of progesterone for women who use estrogen.

On the Horizon

As I've discussed, in the majority of studies on hormones and breast cancer, the researchers failed to differentiate between bioidentical and synthetic hormones. They refer to everything as HRT whether they studied oral or transdermal, carcinogenic, or bioidentical hormones. This makes analyzing the results very confusing. In the next few years, studies making this important distinction will come to fruition. The five-year KEEPS study (Kronos Early Estrogen Prevention Study) started in 2004, and coordinated by the Kronos Longevity Research Institute, a nonprofit clinical research group based in Phoenix, will examine the effects of combined hormone replacement therapy on heart disease prevention in recently menopausal women in two groups. One group will use a transdermal bioidentical estradiol patch along with bioidentical progesterone. The other group will use the oral horse estrogen Premarin with bioidentical progesterone. This study should truly illuminate new findings and reinforce the benefits of bioidentical hormones.

For more information on bioidentical hormones, their safety, and recent research visit the Bioidentical Hormone Initiative at www.bio identicalhormoneinitiative.org, an organization founded by a group of conventionally trained, practicing physicians who have successfully treated patients with bioidentical hormones for many years. On my website, www.femalebraingoneinsane.com, I will keep my readers updated on new and up-coming studies on hormone replacement therapies and their safety.

By now, you have learned how the benefits of taking bioidentical hormones far outweigh the risks. Hormone experts throughout the world have concluded that replacing your hormones is safe, and healthy women going through the first few years of menopause who need HRT to relieve symptoms should have no fears about its use. Making decisions can be confusing and overwhelming at first. Don't despair. For the immediate future, you can make a short-term goal to try bioidentical hormones. Once you start feeling better you will be in a better place emotionally to make long-term decisions.

My most important goal with this book is to offer you hope. There is no need to suffer with your symptoms forever. There is a solution. Bioidentical hormone replacement allows you to enjoy your life and be yourself again. Now you have the opportunity to eliminate all of your unpleasant symptoms. Once you replace the hormones you lack, your emotional well-being will return. It's not about quieting symptoms, it is really about building your body and brain biochemistry back up to strength. Armed with Your Emotional Rescue Plan, you will not only be symptom free, but vivacious and full of life again. There is a light at the end of the tunnel.

Some doctors may not be informed about recent studies and may be on the fence when it comes to bioidentical hormones. Asking your doctor for what you believe is safe and most beneficial for you can be intimidating and overwhelming. To ease your worries and to make it easier for you, I am ending this chapter with a letter that you can bring to your doctor. This letter can be downloaded at www.femalebrain goneinsane.com. The downloaded version includes references to the studies for your doctor's information. The letter is written in professional medical language including scientific evidence supporting your request for bioidentical hormone replacement therapy. You can change it to your specific needs as you desire. Bring this letter and your filled out Emotional Rescue Plan with you when you visit your health care practitioner.

Best of luck to you.

Dear Doctor/Health Care Practitioner,

I am now halfway through a potentially long life, and have found myself without enough of the female hormones needed to remain healthy and vibrant. I am suffering from symptoms clearly related to estrogen deficiency and would like to feel vivacious and full of life again while reducing the risk of osteoporosis, depression, heart attacks, and colon cancer.

I have learned some new and effective treatments to help address my hormone and brain chemistry imbalances and am asking for your help. I just finished reading a book by Mia Lundin, R.N.C., N.P., a nurse practitioner who has in her practice prescribed bioidentical hormones for twenty years. Her book *Female Brain Gone Insane* specifically addresses the delicate dance between the hormones and the brain chemistry, and her treatment plan offers a lot of solid science and practical advice that I would like to follow. Some of her suggestions require your support. I have brought a list of the tests that I would like to have done to evaluate my hormonal status.

Based on resent research (see below) I am not interested in conjugated estrogens (Premarin) or medroxyprogesterone acetate (Provera.) Recent studies indicate that transdermal bioidentical estradiol and oral bioidentical progesterone seems to be the safest and most beneficial combination of hormone replacement therapy today. I do not want to make you uneasy or question your protocols and have included some scientific evidence supporting my decisions.

In 2007, Fournier et al. reported an association between various forms of HRT and the incidence of breast cancer in more than 80,000 postmenopausal women who were followed for more than eight years. Compared with women who had never used any HRT, women who used estrogen only had a non-significant increase of breast cancer. If a synthetic progestin was used in combination with estrogen, the risk for breast cancer increased significantly. However, for women who used bioidentical progesterone in combination with estrogen, the increased risk for breast cancer was eliminated with a significant reduction in breast cancer risk compared with synthetic progestin use. In a previous analysis of more than 50,000 postmenopausal women, Fournier et al. found that the risk for breast cancer was significantly increased if synthetic progestins were used, but was reduced if progesterone was used.

The WHI study clearly proved that Provera (medroxyprogesterone acetate) caused breast cancer and heart disease while Premarin (conjugated estrogens) taken alone showed a decreased incidence of breast cancer and a significant reduction of coronary calcium scores.

The WHI study came to an abrupt halt in July 2002 because the combination of Premarin and Provera also marketed as PremPro showed an increased risk of breast cancer, coronary heart disease, and stroke. Specifically, the study showed women who took the combination of Premarin and Provera had a 24 percent increased risk of breast cancer and an overall 24 percent increased risk of coronary heart disease then those who didn't.

However, what is important to know is that the women who took Premarin without Provera had no increased risk of breast cancer. Also, after five years, the same group of women showed 61 percent less calcified plaque of their coronary arteries compared to the women who took a placebo. Premarin did seem to increase the risk of clotting causing strokes and heart attacks. This risk was amplified when Provera was added. Recent research indicates that when bioidentical estrogen is taken through the skin by patch or cream, this problem is eliminated, and there seems to be no increased risk of clotting.

Several studies, including the Nurses' Health Study and the WHI, showed that those women currently using estrogen replacement therapy or HRT have a significantly lower risk of colorectal cancer. A new finding, published in the January 2009 issue of *Cancer Epidemiology, Biomarkers and Prevention,* found a 17 percent reduced risk of colorectal cancer among women who had at one time used estrogen, a 25 percent reduced risk among women currently using estrogen, and a 26 percent reduced risk among those using estrogen for ten or more years.

The First Global Summit on Menopause-related Issues, held in Zurich on March 29 and 30, 2008, involved forty of the world's leading menopause experts who met to review public perceptions, risks, and benefits of hormone replacement therapy. They looked at four main areas of controversy: cardiovascular health, breast issues, cognition, and bone issues. The summit concluded HRT is safe and that healthy women going through the first few years of the menopause who need HRT to relieve symptoms should have no fears about its use.

The American Association of Clinical Endocrinologists and the North American Menopause Society have also come to similar conclusions.

Further, Amos Pines, president of The International Menopause Society concluded in a 2007 press statement, "Weighing the overall benefits and risks of HT in the younger postmenopausal population clearly favors the use of HT for symptomatic women."

Heart disease is responsible for more deaths in women than all forms of cancer combined and is the most significant health concern for women in the United States today, causing nearly 350,000 deaths each year compared to only 40,000 from breast cancer. Unfortunately, many doctors misconstrued the results of the WHI believing women are better off not taking any hormone replacement therapy. Consequently, many women will needlessly suffer from and be at increased risk for depression, heart disease, stroke, osteoporosis, and colon cancer, while some recent studies indicate that the right type of hormone replacement therapy can significantly reduce the risk of heart disease with no increased risk of breast cancer. Clearly, more studies are needed but until there is evidence to the contrary, it seems that bioidentical hormones should be the preferred method of HRT.

I appreciate you taking the time reading this letter, and I hope I have provided you with enough scientific evidence to support my suggestions for the type hormone replacement therapy I would like to try and look forward to working with you to enhance my health and well-being.

Thank You,

Part Two

Four Steps to Sanity—
Your Emotional
Rescue Plan

Step One: Identify Your Hormonal Phase

As YOU NOW KNOW, your ovaries produce estrogen, progesterone, and some testosterone, hormones you need to keep you healthy and vital. Over time, they produce less and less of these crucial hormones. The complete cessation of hormone production is certainly not an overnight event, but actually takes between ten to fifteen years! That's a long time to go through a variety of emotional and physical ups and downs caused by rising and falling hormones. It is very important to treat your symptoms so you can spend those years living a more vital, happier life.

The ovarian hormone production begins its decline in your mid-to-late thirties and ends with menopause in your early-to-mid fifties. Women in their mid-thirties to mid-fifties are generally not only going through hormonal changes but are under a great deal of external stress, as well. They juggle feisty teenagers, aging parents, the challenges of partnership, and the burdens of work. More stress can contribute to more hormone and brain chemistry imbalances.

Often medical practitioners fail to pay attention to women's hor-

As you read this chapter, make sure you have your Emotional Rescue Plan and pen in hand. Identify your current hormonal phase, and then fill in the treatment best suited for you right now.

mone deficiencies until their symptoms are screaming loud and clear or their periods have finally stopped. That means millions of women are left to suffer as they ride the chaotic emotional hormone roller coaster for years on end, without proper or effective treatment.

This chapter helps you identify your current hormonal phase and suggests bioidentical hormones to help you eliminate unwanted symptoms during your current hormonal phase. Soon you will feel more balanced and in control over your own emotions.

If You Are Taking Birth Control Pills

Often doctors prescribe women birth control pills in an attempt to normalize cycles and symptoms. However, when you take these pills, there is truly nothing normal about your hormones. On the contrary, the potent mixture of synthetic estrogen and synthetic progesterone actually suppress your natural hormones, the very hormones that you need for emotional balance. In addition, the synthetic progesterone in birth control pills can cause a set of emotional symptoms such as agitation, irritability, and rage. If you are suffering from emotional symptoms, you need to *stop* the pills. Of course, you will need to discuss this with your doctor and together find a non-hormonal type of birth control that will still protect you from unwanted pregnancies.

The Four Hormonal Phases

As your ovarian hormones decline, you will transition through four major hormonal phases. Each of the four phases has its own set of potential emotional and physical symptoms and solutions. Some women just slide through these transitions without many symptoms while others encounter all kinds of emotional and physical challenges.

Review your Monthly Symptom Tracker and read below to determine your hormonal phase.

- Phase 1: Normal Hormones—The Steady State

  Your emotional symptoms are not cyclic. Of course, we all feel a little different from day to day, but when you are in this phase, your symptoms do not increase drastically before your expected period, meaning you do not suffer from PMS.

- Phase 2: PMS—The Cyclical Crazy Zone

  The symptoms in this phase always occur before menses and generally last from a few days to two full weeks. They can cause a great deal of short-term discomfort, but distress ends once menses begins.

- Phase 3: Perimenopause—The Irrational Erratic Zone

  The symptoms in this phase tend to be erratic and occur before your period as well, but do not end once menses begin. Symptoms tend to continue for another week at least.

- Phase 4: Menopause and Postmenopause—The Flat Zone

  The symptoms in this phase are pretty much the same day after day. They are not erratic anymore, and of course, you do not experience menses.

- Women with Hysterectomies

  Women who have had hysterectomies with or with the removal of their ovaries require a unique treatment plan.

Let's review all of the phases in detail so you can fully understand each phase and correctly identify your current phase.

Phase 1: Normal Hormones—The Steady State

Before focusing on your particular hormonal imbalances, take a look at what your hormones look like in a normal menstrual cycle.

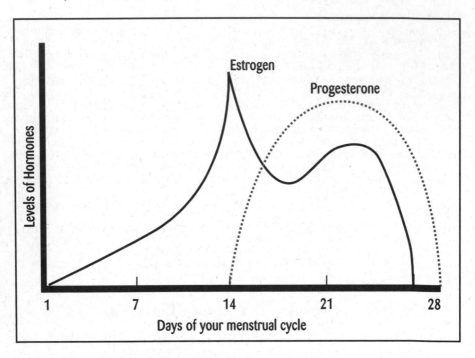

During a normal menstrual cycle:

- Estrogen is normal. This means it spikes mid-cycle and tells the ovary to let go of an egg (ovulation).
- The site where the egg emerges becomes a little factory for the production of progesterone.
- Progesterone is produced when you ovulate.
- The progesterone spikes to its highest level around day 21 to 24 (the best days in the cycle to check your progesterone levels).

- If you don't get pregnant this month, your progesterone drops back to its lowest level right before menstruation.
- After ovulation, your estrogen level begins to drop and then hits its lowest level during menses.
- You have normal, regular menstrual cycles, bleeding every 28–32 days.

Some women whose hormones are normal still experience uncomfortable emotional symptoms such as anxiety or depression throughout the month. Are you one of these women? If so, you are not suffering from PMS because there is no cyclic pattern to your distress. You do not have a hormonal imbalance, but you do have a brain chemistry imbalance—possibly from nutritional deficiencies and stress. I have found that many women in your situation respond really well to nutritional treatments that support your body to feel emotionally well. If this is your profile, please turn directly to Step Two: Discover your Emotional Type and follow through the Four Steps to Sanity in Your Emotional Rescue Plan.

Phase 2: PMS—The Cyclical Crazy Zone

As you age, the first hormone that declines in your body is actually progesterone. In your mid-to-late thirties, your progesterone level drops as anovulatory cycles—meaning ovulation does not take place—become more prevalent. Even if ovulation still occurs, progesterone levels are not at their optimum levels. This decline in progesterone causes a variety of PMS symptoms. In my office, I often hear, "I feel so much rage and irritability about a week or so before my period. Once my period starts, it is like a switch is turned off and all my symptoms instantly go away."

Studies show that symptoms of PMS, such as anxiety, irritability, and rage are associated with sharp declines in circulating progesterone levels, leading to low levels of GABA or a decline of GABA receptors (the calming neurotransmitter). Other studies consider the neurotransmitter serotonin as a key factor involved in the development of symptoms of PMS. Biochemically, patients with PMS symptoms have lower levels of serotonin in their blood and urine during the premenstrual phase of their menstrual cycle. They lack the chemical that can give them a sense of calm or well-being.

Meet Monica

Monica is thirty-nine years old and a mother of two young children. She is married and a stay at home mom. When she first came to see me she said, "Most of the month I feel fine. I am happy, in control of my emotions, and enjoy spending time with my kids. About seven to ten days before my period, everything changes. I get agitated, have no tolerance, and yell like a crazy woman. I truly feel like I am insane and begin to feel like I had better not be alone with the children or else. It is like I have lost control over my own behavior. I hate myself for acting this way, and I feel like I am failing big time at being a mom. When my husband comes home, I scream at him too. He looks at me in shock, and often says, 'Why are you acting this way? You were just fine a couple of days ago.' I wonder too."

I asked Monica how she felt once her period started. "All of a sudden I feel like my old self again. I'm patient, kind, and even lovable! Of course, then I feel guilty about how I acted and vow that next month I will do better. Of course, next month rolls along and there I go

Mia's Mantra

You are not going crazy

again! I feel like a complete failure as a mom and a wife. Please help me." I told Monica she was suffering from classic PMS and recommended the following rescue treatment: I started her on bioidentical progesterone to normalize her progesterone, and nutritional support including 5-HTP, a B6 complex, and magnesium to increase her serotonin level. I also recommended she drink my morning protein smoothie (see recipe on page 129).

She returned six weeks later. "I can't believe how much you have helped me. Last month I felt so much better. I was kinder to my children, I felt in control over my emotions, and just wasn't angry or crazy anymore." With a smile on her face she added, "My husband also said to tell you 'thank you!'"

How do you know that you are in the PMS phase and not going through the next phase known as perimenopause? The big clue lies in your emotional symptoms. The symptoms of true PMS only appear between ovulation (midcycle) and the onset of your menses (bleeding.) Some women only have symptoms for a few days before their period, while others suffer for two full weeks. The symptoms tend to escalate the closer to the period you get. Once your menstrual flow starts, the symptoms magically disappear and you are back to your old self again. Your mood can improve in a matter of hours after starting your period. Once you hit perimenopause, this distinct switch from horrible symptoms to feeling just fine does not seem to happen.

Emotional symptoms of PMS you might experience one to two weeks before your period:

- Irritability
- Rage

- Feeling overwhelmed
- Feeling revved up
- Depression
- Anxiety
- Mood swings
- Reduced self-esteem

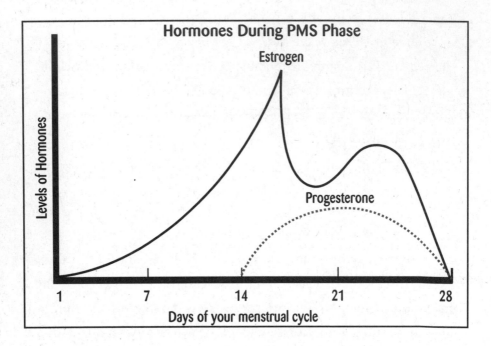

During the PMS phase, your period occurs regularly—every 28 to 32 days—although it might be a little heavier than in previous years.

- Progesterone is lower than it used to be in the normal menstrual cycle.
- Some months the ovaries produce more progesterone than others. This is the reason your symptoms are sometimes worse.

Your Emotional Rescue Plan for PMS

The recommended hormone to alleviate symptoms during PMS is progesterone. By using bioidentical progesterone you will raise the low levels of progesterone in the premenstrual phase of your cycle, creating a calming effect. Ah yes, relief! This will reduce agitation and anxiety. Use the progesterone only during the days of your cycle as recommended. It is not to be used all month long. Try the protocol on page 82 for a few months and pay attention. Do your symptoms improve? Use your Monthly Symptom Tracker as a tool. Think positive! If you do not feel much improvement in one to two months, see a health care practitioner who specializes in hormonal issues and bioidentical hormone replacement therapy.

Phase 3: Perimenopause—The Irrational Erratic Zone

The majority of women that come to see me are in the perimenopausal phase. This is the time women feel the most emotional distress. I can't tell you how many patients walk into my office and announce:

- "I feel like I am totally out of control."
- "I cannot predict who I'll be from day to day."
- "I'm really going insane."

Perimenopause is the hormonal transition that takes place before a woman stops menstruating. It is a challenging time as perimenopause often lasts for years on end, and your estrogen level fluctuates from high to low, and back to high again. This creates a set of inconsistent and highly distressful physical and emotional symptoms and behaviors.

During perimenopause, your calming hormone progesterone is also at a lower level than normal. You may still have a monthly period, but it comes a few days closer together with a heavier flow than in the past often with blood clots. Often doctors prescribe birth control pills to lessen the heavy, clotty, or more frequent periods. They may also recommend antidepressants to address emotional distress. Some doctors even recommend a D & C (dilatation and curettage) or hysterectomy to alleviate heavy bleeding, while never presenting the option of bioidentical progesterone therapy. Taking bioidentical progesterone often eliminates the heavy bleeding without requiring surgery.

In perimenopause estrogen fluctuates up and down. Every time it drops, your brain neurotransmitter serotonin also drops. This is the neurotransmitter that gives you a feeling of peace and calm. So, your serotonin drops, causing symptoms such as irritability, anxiety, insomnia, and low libido. Along with the drop comes a craving for carbohydrates and alcohol.

When serotonin drops, the "fight or flight" neurotransmitter norepinephrine suddenly spikes. This may cause nervousness, a pounding heart, interrupted sleep, upset stomach, and sometimes high blood pressure. The body perceives this as stress and so the adrenal glands release a hormone called cortisol. Cortisol blocks T3 production (the active very important thyroid hormone), and high cortisol also increases the level of insulin.

So you end up with a lower thyroid, which slows down your metabolism, and high levels of the fat storing hormone, insulin. Insulin takes the sugar from your carbohydrate and alcohol consumption and stores it as fat. This results in weight gain, especially around your middle. The cortisol (adrenal hormone) also blocks your estrogen receptors so estrogen can no longer enter the cells. You are without the estrogen you need, and the vicious cycle continues again and again!

Meet Brenda

Brenda is forty-three-year-old mom with a thirteen-year-old daughter and sixteen-year-old son. Until a few months ago, she had regular twenty-eight day menstrual cycles. In the past, she suffered from PMS symptoms (feeling angry and out of control) a couple of days before her period began, but as soon as she flowed she felt normal again.

Now her periods are coming a little closer together (23 to 25 days instead of 28), are heavy with some clotting, and she is bleeding more days than before. She complains of intermittent night sweats and hot flashes. Her breasts are tender much of the time and she feels that her PMS symptoms are more intense, and are accompanied by rage and irritability. She emphasizes that when her period starts she does not get the kind of relief from her symptoms that she used to. Now she suffers from crying spells, insomnia, and extreme fatigue during the week of menses.

Brenda lives in an irrational and erratic zone, swinging from crying to rage to guilt. Her gynecologist did not diagnose her as perimenopausal, but said a hysterectomy may be in order if her periods become much heavier. He also thought her emotional problems might be from depression or bipolar disorder, and he referred her to a psychiatrist for evaluation. Brenda began taking an antidepressant, but claimed her anxiety and insomnia actually increased. There was no change in her menstrual cycle.

I spoke with Brenda about her symptoms and performed an exam. Based on her recent history of heavy clotty periods, shorter cycles, and the lack of relief of symptoms once her period began, I determined she was perimenopausal.

Although she was quite distraught, I knew from experience that I could normalize her cycle, and she would feel much better once she began her program of using bioidentical progesterone. After only one month on her treatment plan, which also included nutritional supplements for her emotional type, Brenda returned to her follow-up visit with a smile on her face. She was amazed at how quickly she responded to the treatment. Her menstrual cycle was now back to twenty-eight days, her periods were normal, with no clotting, and her days were filled with less anxiety and more peace.

It's important to understand that the relationship between Brenda's hormones and her brain chemistry created her mood, and that treating her with progesterone alone would not take care of her discordant symptoms. In addition, she needed nutritional supplements to normalize her brain chemistry.

Perimenopausal Symptoms Speak Loudly

So, I ask you again, how do you know that you are in the perimenopausal phase and still not in the PMS phase? The answer lies in your emotional symptoms: they do not go away when you start bleeding. Instead of feeling cranky and irritable and then flowing and feeling good again, your symptoms hang around, even during your menses. Many women tell me, "I only feel like I used to, and that means good, maybe one week a month." This good week is usually the second week of the monthly cycle, day seven through fourteen from the first day of bleeding, when the symptoms quiet down and your hormones are more balanced. One week is not enough!

Here are some symptoms you might experience. Some appear only one to two weeks before your period, others the week you bleed, while some overlap. Do you have any of the following? If so, you are probably perimenopausal and should follow the recommended plan starting on page 80.

Perimenopausal symptoms you might experience one to two weeks before your period:

- Irritability
- Rage
- Feeling overwhelmed
- Feeling revved
- Depression
- Anxiety
- Mood swings
- Reduced self-esteem
- Hot flashes and night sweats

Perimenopausal symptoms you might experience the week you bleed:

- Fatigue
- Sadness
- Crying easily
- Insomnia

Menstrual Changes During Perimenopause:

- Your periods tend to come closer together (21- to 24-day cycle instead of 28- to 30-day cycle) but can still be regular.
- Heavier bleeding, sometimes clotting, sometimes more cramping.
- Symptoms and bleeding patterns change from month to month as hormone levels vary.
- Progesterone is now lower than in the PMS phase.
- Estrogen is often high and erratic as it attempts to compensate for low progesterone levels. Each time the estrogen level drops, it causes emotional symptoms as well as hot flashes, headaches, and night sweats.

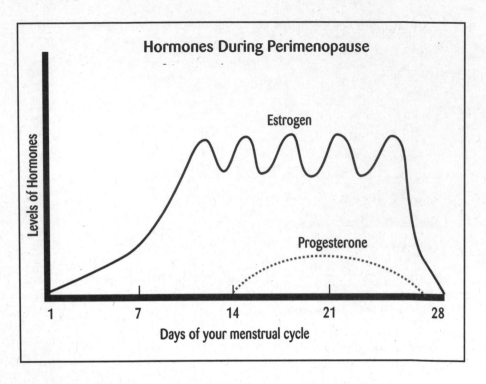

Your Emotional Rescue Plan for PMS and Perimenopause

The key to treating your PMS and perimenopausal symptoms is progesterone. I use both progesterone capsules and creams for women in either the PMS or perimenopausal phase. Oral progesterone tends to be more sedating, and I recommend it only for women who are very anxious and revved up. Try the following protocol for a few months to see if your symptoms improve.

Bioidentical progesterone will raise the low progesterone levels and create a calming effect, which will reduce agitation and anxiety. It will also balance the high and erratic estrogen in perimenopause bringing it back to normal, while normalizing menstruation resulting in less bleeding and clotting. The progesterone should eliminate the emotional symptoms you experience during the rest of your cycle as well. If you

do not feel much better after following my recommendations, see a health care practitioner who
specializes in hormonal issues and bioidentical hormone replacement therapy. You might
be close to menopause and in need of bioidentical estrogen as well.

You should listen to your symptoms, but if you wish to test your hormones to confirm you are in the perimenopause phase, see pages 97 and 98.

The healthier you are, the longer your
ovaries will function. High stress, lack of nutrients, and a sedentary lifestyle tend to push women
into perimenopause earlier than if their life was more
balanced. In addition to my recommendations for bioidentical progesterone, nutritional supplements, and lifestyle changes, I often rec
ommend acupuncture for my perimenopausal patients.

Current research shows that acupuncture treatment has a positive
influence on the production and circulation of hormones in the body.
Acupuncture provides nourishment to the internal organs, including
the ovaries. If there is a disruption in the flow of blood and energy to
the ovaries, acupuncture can regulate the flow and energy to restore
hormonal balance and reduce perimenopausal symptoms. Many of my
perimenopausal patients who sought help from acupuncturists actually
shortened the length of their perimenopausal phases, thereby reducing
the unpleasant symptoms of irritability, depression, and anxiety often
associated with this hormonal phase.

Try acupuncture in addition to following my nutritional advice, supplement recommendations, and stress-relieving techniques in Steps
Two, Three, and Four to gain the greatest benefit.

Progesterone

PRODUCT	HOW TO USE
Over-the-counter Emerita Progesterone Topical Cream or any of the progesterone creams recommended at www.femalebraingoneinsane.com. If you have your own source, make sure it contains 20 mg of USP progesterone per gram.	¼ teaspoon *(equals 1 gram)* twice daily during days 16–28 of your menstrual cycle. Rub the cream into the skin of inner arms or inner thighs.
Prescription Compounded Micronized Progesterone Cream *(this is the actual name).***	• 16 mg/mL—if it comes in a syringe for dosing. • Use 1 mL twice daily, days 16–28 of your menstrual cycle. Rub the cream in to inner arms or inner thighs. • 16 mg/gram if it comes in a jar. • Use 1 gram or ¼ tsp twice daily, days 16–28 of your menstrual cycle. • Rub the cream in to inner arms or inner thighs.
Compounded oral-micronized progesterone capsules.**	• 50–100 mg by mouth, twice daily, days 16–28 of your menstrual cycle.*
Prometrium® caplets*** *(available at most pharmacies).*	• 50–100 mg by mouth. Twice daily, days 16–28 of your menstrual cycle.

*When you count your days, note that day one is your first day of bleeding.
**See Resources for Sanity to find compounding pharmacies.
***I don't usually recommend Prometrium because it is compounded with peanut oil, and many women are allergic to peanuts.

Progesterone cream can be purchase online or at health food stores. Choose one of the high quality products I recommend or ask your health care practitioner to prescribe one. Then fill in Step 1 on Your Emotional Rescue Plan.

Record shifts and changes in your symptoms on your Monthly Symptom Tracker as you use the progesterone and adjust the amount according to the recommendations below. Trust yourself on this one. When you apply the right amount of progesterone you will feel better with no annoying side effects, and your menstrual cycle should normalize back to twenty-eight to thirty-two days.

Using Too Much Progesterone:

- You may feel increased cramping and bloating with your period.
- You may feel dopey (progesterone is a natural tranquilizer) with symptoms such as tiredness, grogginess, and depression.

Using Too Little Progesterone:

- You may still experience heavy, clotty periods.
- You continue to have symptoms of irritability, agitation, anxiety.

Phase 4: Menopause—The Flat Zone

Menopause signifies the time in your life when your menstrual cycle ends. The word comes from the Greek word *mens,* meaning monthly, and *pausis,* meaning cessation. A part of your natural aging process, menopause occurs when your ovaries produce very low levels of the hormones of estrogen and progesterone. You are not ovulating anymore so you are no longer able to become pregnant. The average age for menopause is fifty-two. However, menopause can normally occur anytime between the ages of forty-two and fifty-six. At first, your periods come months apart, and eventually they cease. Likely, you are in menopause when you have not had a period for a full year. However, some women still have a few periods per year even after menopause.

In the February 2009 edition of *O, The Oprah Magazine,* Oprah

Winfrey tells how she felt out of kilter and had issues that she suspected were hormone related for nearly two years. After finally seeking help, Winfrey's hormone specialist told her that her hormonal tank was empty and gave her a prescription for bioidentical estrogen. "After one day on bioidentical estrogen, I felt the veil lift," Winfrey said. "After three days, the sky was bluer, my brain was no longer fuzzy, and my memory was sharper. I was literally singing and had a skip in my step."

Meet Francine

Francine is a forty-nine-year-old, stay-at-home mom who has been married for twenty-five years—and until six months ago, happily so. Before having children, she worked as a nurse. Now, her nineteen-year-old son is in college and her seventeen-year-old daughter is a senior in high school.

Francine cried while she told me her story. "I used to be such a together person, happy and easy going. I got things done in a wink, loved being a mom and a wife, but for the last six months everything has changed. I can't seem to be able to feel joy anymore. I am panicked about my daughter leaving for college in a year. Then what? I have been a mom for so long, I don't know what my purpose is anymore. I cry for nothing, I can't sleep, I am exhausted all the time, and my brain feels like it belongs to somebody else. I used to love my husband, but I am not so sure I want to stay with him. I have no desire for sex and feel repulsed when he touches me. I look out the window and the world seems to lack color or delight."

When I asked Francine about her periods, she told me she has only had one period within the last four months and it was very light. On her exam, her vaginal tissue was very pale and thin looking, consistent with low estrogen, meaning menopause.

I started Francine on a bioidentical estrogen patch and cyclic bioidentical progesterone. I also started her on the Basic Supplement Program. When she came back to see me in a month, she said, "Mia, I am not kidding, within hours after I applied the estrogen patch to my tummy, the world around me just changed. I felt an instant lift and so much happier. Within a couple of nights, I was able to sleep again and started feeling more energetic."

When I asked her about her relationship with her husband, she said, "What do you mean? It is great. I love him, and we are having a blast. We just went away for a weekend together, had great sex and good food. I am considering going back to nursing part time, and I am actually excited about the prospect of having the house to ourselves with our kids going away to college."

This story is true; it is not fiction, and it demonstrates how drastically symptoms can improve with bioidentical hormones. When the body gets what it is screaming for, in this case estrogen and progesterone, it comes back into balance, and the mind feels at ease and happy again. I can't count how many women I have seen in my office who couldn't stand their husbands or significant others and were ready for a divorce. I always would tell them to wait. Don't do anything yet. Try the treatment, and then let's talk more about that at your next visit. The next month, their divorce plan was usually forgotten, as was the case with Francine.

The Symptoms of Menopause

So how do you know you are out of the perimenopausal phase and in menopause? The symptoms of perimenopause and menopause can be very similar and hard to differentiate. You can also go back and forth between perimenopause and menopause. Blood levels of estrogen fluctuate a lot in both perimenopause and early menopause, and blood tests are not very useful when attempting to diagnose menopause. The blood test for follicular stimulating hormone (FSH) can give you an indication, but recent research indicates it not very reliable.

The best way to diagnose menopause is through your emotional symptoms. My menopausal patients often say:

- "I feel flat, and the world does not seem to be in color anymore."
- "I feel dry like cardboard, I look like cardboard, and my brain feels like cardboard."
- "I don't care anymore, and I don't care that I don't care."

A common symptom in menopause is a "lump in the throat" feeling, where you have become very sensitive to all things and may begin crying at the drop of a pin. In addition, during menopause your symptoms tend to be more consistent than during perimenopause. Your feelings of sadness or lethargy remain with you day after day.

Common menopausal symptoms:

- Dry eyes and skin
- Fatigue
- Hot flashes
- Insomnia
- Itchy skin
- Joint pain
- Weight gain—especially in the middle
- Pounding heart
- Skipping heart beats
- "Creepy crawly skin," which feels like bugs are crawling on your skin
- Sadness

- Mood swings
- Crying spells
- Night sweats
- Depression
- Difficulty focusing
- Irritability
- Anxiety
- Pale vaginal tissue
- Vaginal dryness
- Short-term memory problems
- You do not menstruate anymore or only rarely

Observing your symptoms and sometimes just a trial treatment with bioidentical estrogen and or progesterone or a cycle of progesterone only (as recommended for the perimenopausal phase) will give you a good indication of your hormonal phase.

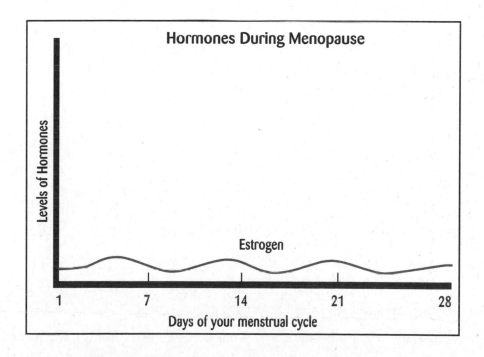

During Menopause:

- You no longer ovulate and are not producing any progesterone.
- The estrogen level is very low throughout the month.

Hysterectomy With or Without Ovaries Removed

Some gynecologists recommend hysterectomies as the first line of treatment for irregular or heavy bleeding in perimenopausal or menopausal women. I have seen hundreds of patients who opted for hysterectomies on the advice of their doctors. The doctors were familiar with the surgical procedures, but they had no knowledge of or training in the follow-up treatment of replacing hormones.

If you have had a complete hysterectomy (when both the uterus and ovaries are removed) your body goes from experiencing relatively normal hormonal levels to complete hormonal bankruptcy in less than an hour. This can have catastrophic consequences in women sensitive to hormonal shifts, causing extreme emotional symptoms of anxiety and depression. After a complete hysterectomy, you need bioidentical estrogen, and probably testosterone, to start feeling normal.

Although most women are told they don't need progesterone after a hysterectomy, recent research indicates that women who took bioidentical progesterone in addition to estrogen had less breast cancer. Therefore, I often recommend the use of progesterone even for women who have had a hysterectomy. Also, many of my patients feel better once progesterone is added as they benefit from the calming and diuretic effects progesterone provides. Women with simple hysterectomies (removal of the uterus with the ovaries left in tact) also often suffer symptoms from hormonal imbalances, probably due to some damage or reduced blood supply to the ovaries after surgery. I always recommend that women who suffer symptoms after a hysterectomy have their hormones checked to see if progesterone and estrogen may help them.

Meet Barbara

Barbara was forty-seven with two children, thirteen and seventeen years old. She had been happily married for nineteen years. Other than experiencing the blues for a couple of weeks after her second child, she denied any history of depression or anxiety. She used to have regular menses until her mid-forties when her period became very heavy with clots. She also started to suffer from menstrual cramps, which she had never had before.

At her last annual exam, her gynecologist diagnosed uterine fibroids (benign growths of the uterus) and determined that Barbara's emotional symptoms were due to them. Her doctor said Barbara's uterus was the size of a three-month pregnancy and recommended a hysterectomy with the removal of her ovaries. In addition, the doctor told her that the procedure was fairly simple and that she would completely recover within four to six weeks. Barbara received counseling about the benefits of estrogen replacement therapy after surgery to prevent common symptoms such as hot flashes, night sweats, and vaginal dryness. No one even suggested that mood changes could also be a real and possible postsurgery symptom.

After her hysterectomy, Barbara took the prescription derived from horse estrogen called Premarin. At first she felt tired, but otherwise fine. Four weeks later, Barbara started to feel anxious almost daily, as well as bloated. In addition, her breasts were tender and her bra size had increased from a B- to a D-cup.

Two weeks later, Barbara woke up in the middle of the night sweating and shaking. She felt like she could not breathe and was drowning in fear. Barbara had her husband call 911. She arrived at the emergency room, and the doctor said she was having a panic attack. Barbara went back to her gynecologist, who had performed her hysterectomy, for an evaluation of her hormonal status. By then, she had not slept for three nights and told him, "I feel like I am going crazy, I am losing it!"

Not educated on the estradiol-serotonin connection, Barbara's gynecologist referred her to a psychiatrist who prescribed the antianxiety drug Xanax, and the antidepressant Prozac. Both the gynecologist and the psychiatrist failed to recognize her symptoms were from a hormonal imbalance. By the time I saw her, she felt somewhat better and could sleep for four to five hours a night—probably because of the prescriptions. She said she had less anxiety, but she just did not feel like her old self. She said, "I feel like I am walking in a fog, and I am tired all the time. My sex drive is completely gone, and I am unable to achieve orgasm. Is this how I will feel for the rest of my life?"

I explained that her initial symptoms of anxiety and panic were most likely due to a hormonal imbalance. Her estrogen, progesterone, and testosterone producing glands—the ovaries—had been removed, and yet she was prescribed non-bioidentical estrogen only. Contrary to what most doctors seem to believe, some women who have had their ovaries removed do need more than just estrogen replacement. They need all three hormones balanced in order to feel harmonious.

We have receptors for all three hormones throughout the body—not just in the uterus and ovaries—but in the brain, bones, and skin. These receptors still need stimulation even though the uterus and ovaries have been removed! Barbara had started on Premarin, which causes numerous side effects such as bloating and breast tenderness. However, she was not offered progesterone or testosterone.

I recommended Barbara stop her Premarin. In its place, I started her on a bioidentical estrogen patch, nightly bioidentical progesterone, and a small dose of testosterone. The bioidentical progesterone acts as

You should listen to your symptoms, but if you wish to test your hormones to confirm you are in the menopause phase, see pages 97 and 98.

a diuretic and has a calming effect. It also seems to help with insomnia. Testosterone replacement will increase the feeling of well-being and give back a sex drive.

Two weeks after Barbara started on my protocol, I tested her hormones, and they were all within normal range. Barbara was so amazed that she felt calm and content again. She was able to stop taking Xanax right away, and during the following month, she was slowly weaned off her Prozac. Barbara began her life again, in balance and at ease.

Emotional Rescue Plan for Menopause and Women with Hysterectomies

Menopause requires a combination of bioidentical estrogen, progesterone, and often testosterone to make you feel better. Bioidentical estrogen is the key to eliminating your symptoms during menopause. It will take you from flat to functional and then to feeling good. However, you cannot purchase it over the counter. That means you need to work with your health care practitioner so that you can get a prescription.

Although estrogen is a very beneficial hormone, it can cause problems if not used in the correct and recommended amounts. Your health care practitioner must monitor you over time with occasional blood tests to ensure absorption and normal levels. As your estrogen level builds, you will feel more at ease. Fluctuating levels of estrogen can cause night sweats, hot flashes, mood swings, and head aches. Therefore, estrogen should be used every day of the month. Progesterone can be used daily (continuous therapy) or twelve days out of the month (cyclic therapy). If you still have a uterus, always use the estrogen with bioidentical progesterone to lower the risk of uterine cancer. The risk of uterine cancer is increased five-fold if estrogen is used without progesterone.

In general, I start my patients on the cyclic therapy beginning with estrogen by itself for one to two weeks. Then I'll add progesterone to the mix to see how they feel with the combination. With cyclic therapy, monthly menstrual bleeding can occur. Some health care practitioners prefer non-cyclic, but daily treatment. I have found daily treatment works better once the patient is at least three to five years into menopause, because starting continuous therapy too early tends to cause annoying break-through bleeding and spotting.

Estradiol to the Rescue

Your ovaries make three different types of estrogen: estrone (E1), estradiol (E2), and estriol (E3). Estradiol is the estrogen that really makes a difference when it comes to improving your mood. The ovaries often continue to make some estrone after menopause. I also use estriol cream, but only for vaginal dryness.

The biochemical name for estradiol is 17ß-estradiol, which is what you will read in the package inserts or on the label of your estrogen. Bioidentical estradiol comes in pills, patches, creams, sprays, and gels. All forms of bioidentical estradiol are available through regular pharmacies by prescription only. In some cases, the capsules, creams, and gels are compounded, which means the pharmacist hand-mixes the ingredients to fit the unique requirements of the prescription. Prescriptions may be compounded to omit a nonessential ingredient that the patient is allergic to, or to obtain the exact dose needed. However, a hormone does not have to be compounded by a pharmacy to be bioidentical. The raw material in both compounded and prepared prescriptions is the same.

I prefer my patients use transdermal (through the skin via cream, gel, or patch) whenever possible. Recent research indicates that oral (by mouth) estradiol may have some risks that transdermal estradiol does not. For example:

- Oral estrogen can increase the risk of stroke, high blood pressure, heart attack, and blood clots.
- Any estrogen taken orally goes through the liver and stimulates binding proteins for thyroid, testosterone, adrenal hormones, and growth hormone. It can reduce the availability of these hormones to the cells.
- Oral estradiol will increase inflammation, including C-reactive protein (CRP), which increases the risk of heart disease.
- The liver first metabolizes oral estrogen and then changes it into a metabolite of estradiol, which, biochemically, does not look like the beneficial estradiol anymore. It is no longer "the right key for the right keyhole."
- Oral estrogen increases insulin resistance.

Estradiol cannot be purchased over the counter. Your health care practitioner must prescribe it. After receiving a prescription, record it in Step One of Your Emotional Rescue Plan.

Transdermal Estradiol

Name	Delivery method	Dosing
Vivelle Dot	Transdermal patch	Twice weekly
Climara	Transdermal patch	Once weekly
EstroGel	Topical gel	1-4 pumps daily
Estrasorb	Topical cream	1-2 packets daily
Divigel	Transdermal gel	1 pack daily
Menostar	Transdermal patch	Weekly
Eva Mist	Transdermal spray	1–3 sprays daily

Compounded Transdermal Estradiol

Name	Dosing
Estradiol gel 1-4mg/mL	1 mL twice daily to inner arms or inner thighs.

Ask your health care practitioner to prescribe the right dose and the best type of bioidentical estradiol for you. Then, record it in Step One of Your Emotional Rescue Plan. Note: If you use too much estrogen, you may feel jittery, amped up, bloated, or breast tenderness (a really good clue) and may need a lower dose. If you still suffer from a variety of menopausal symptoms you probably need a higher dose. In either case, talk with your doctor, and ask for an adjustment to your prescription.

Be aware, the following are not bioidentical hormones and should not be used:

• Brand names such as Premarin, Activella Angeliq, PremPro, Premphase, FemHRT, Combi Patch, and Climara Pro.

• All birth control pills.

• Synthetic progesterone, known as progestin, such as Provera.

Add Bioidentical Progesterone to Your Rescue Plan

If you are menopausal and using estrogen, you need to use a bioidentical progesterone as well to prevent a build-up of the uterine lining that can lead to uterine cancer. My preferred type of progesterone for women using estrogen is the oral progesterone. Add progesterone within a month of starting estrogen. Below are examples of both commercially made and compounded preparations. Oral bioidentical progesterone cannot be purchased over the counter. Your health care practitioner must prescribe it.

Ask your doctor to prescribe one of the following bioidentical progesterones. Then, record it in Step One of Your Emotional Rescue Plan.

Bioidentical Progesterone

Name	Delivery method	Dosing
Prometrium*	Oral gel capsule	• 100 mg by mouth twice daily for 12 days/month, or • 200 mg at bedtime for 12 nights/month, or • 100 mg every night. * Be aware that if you have peanut allergies this product contains peanut oil
Prochieve	Vaginal gel	Supplied in a 4 or 8 percent concentration in disposable, single-use applicators. Each 1.125 grams of gel delivers either 45 mg or 90 mg of progesterone. Suggested use is every other night for six nights per month.
Compounded Micronized Progesterone	Oral capsules	• 100 mg twice daily for 12 days/month, or • 200 mg at bedtime for 12 nights/month, or • 100 mg every night

Note: These are my usual recommendations only. Your health care practitioner will determine the right dose and type of bioidentical progesterone best for you.

Testosterone

You may not know it, but testosterone is not only important for men, but also for women. As we age our testosterone levels decline. Excessive stress, some medications, contraceptives, and surgical removal of the ovaries can lower our testosterone. Low testosterone leads to symptoms including loss of libido, thinning skin, vaginal dryness, and loss of bone and muscle mass, depression, and memory lapses. Some of my patients do not feel quite right until we gently raise their testosterone to normal levels.

Common symptoms of low testosterone:

• Low sex drive
• Fatigue
• "Flatness" of mood
• Low energy
• Difficulty focusing

Common symptoms of too much testosterone:

• Aggressiveness
• Increased body hair
• Oily skin
• Agitation
• Over-active sex drive

Testosterone cannot be purchased over the counter. Your health care practitioner must prescribe it. After receiving a prescription, record it in Step One of Your Emotional Rescue Plan.

Bioidentical Testosterone

Name	Delivery method	Dosing
Testosterone gel or cream *(By compounding pharmacies)*	Transdermal	0.5–3 mg daily Use on inner arms or thighs
Testosterone capsules *(By compounding pharmacies)*	Oral	0.5–3 mg daily

How to Test Your Hormone Levels

I believe your symptoms are a better indicator of your hormonal phase than any testing because hormone levels vary from day to day and month to month. If you want to have your hormone levels tested anyway and still get your period, have your estrogen, progesterone, and testosterone checked on days twenty-one through twenty-four of your menstrual cycle, and FSH should be checked on days three through five of your menstrual cycle. First day of bleeding is day one.

Saliva Tests

The following laboratories have saliva test kits available for purchase and can provide you with a hormone analysis. Each lab will provide you with their reference values (normal levels).

Body balance at www.bodybalance.com

• Female Health Check (estrogen, progesterone, testosterone).

ZRT Laboratory at www.zrtlab.com

• Saliva test: Hormone Profile I (estradiol, progesterone, testosterone, DHEA-S, and morning cortisol).

• Blood Spot: (Blood spot is a simple finger prick test followed by placing blood drops on a filter card. The card is then sent to the laboratory for analysis.) Female Hormone Profile, (estradiol, progesterone, testosterone, SHBG [sex hormone binding globulin]).

Laboratory Blood Tests

You can either ask your doctor for the following tests or you can order your own blood tests at MyMedLab.com or through Life Extension Foundation; (lef.org) see pages 211–212 for more information. The websites will provide you with a list of blood draw stations throughout the country. Once you receive your test results, you and your health care practitioner can review them and determine a treatment plan.

Blood Test Measurements:

- FSH level: This is a blood test that should be drawn 3 to 5 days after the first day of your menstrual bleeding. Normal FSH day 3 value is 3–10 mU/mL. FSH levels above 10–12 mU/mL indicate that your ovaries are starting to produce fewer hormones. This indicates that you are in perimenopause. FSH levels about 30–40 or above usually signal that you are in menopause.

- Progesterone level: This is also a blood test and should be drawn day 21 to 24 of the menstrual cycle. Normal progesterone level should be around 20–28 ng/mL at that time of the cycle.

- Testosterone level: This is also a blood test and should be drawn day 21 to 24 of the menstrual cycle. Many commercial laboratories list normal serum testosterone levels up to 70 to 80 ng/dL; however, most of my patients feel their best if their level is somewhere between 40–80 ng/dL.

By now, you should know your current hormonal phase and the best combination of bioidentical hormones that is right for you. Hormonal balance provides the infrastructure required for well-being. With the right hormone combination, you have the solid foundation to build a happy and rewarding life. Rest assured, your misery will soon become a distant memory.

Step Two: Discover Your Emotional Type

Aʟʟ OF US FEEL SAD OR ANXIOUS at certain points in our lives. Fleeting feelings of sadness and disappointment or nervousness and discomfort are perfectly normal, especially during difficult times. You may also experience occasional sleep problems as well as bouts of panic or fear. If these disruptive feelings do not disappear within approximately two weeks, you may be suffering from an imbalance of your brain chemistry. Your symptoms will tell which brain chemical you lack and what amino acids and other supplements you need to take to rebalance your brain chemistry and find relief. Even though your symptoms may make you feel like you are falling apart, don't worry: you will pull yourself together again, and soon. I see women with a variety of symptoms in my practice, but most of them fit one of the following three Emotional Types:

- Revved Up and Anxious
- I Can't Get Off The Couch
- The Combination

As you read this chapter, you will determine your Emotional Type based on your symptoms and learn the exact supplements to take to best support it. If you prefer to have your brain chemistry levels tested, your health care practitioner will need to order the tests for you. However, your symptoms are an excellent gauge. Make sure to use Your Emotional Rescue Plan worksheet to fill in your Emotional Type and your supplement regimen.

After you learn to identify your Emotional Type, you can read the short profiles of women who felt the way you do and what treatment protocols they followed to find balance again. There is a treatment protocol for each of the three Emotional Types, consisting of combinations of amino acids, vitamins, and supplements. Copy the appropriate recommendations for your Emotional Type on to your Emotional Rescue Plan and you've completed the legwork for Step Two. This approach is not mysterious. It is direct and makes sense to supply your body with exactly what it needs to keep you happy and balanced!

Which Emotional Type Are You?

Refer to your Monthly Symptom Tracker to see the patterns of your physical and emotional symptoms. Answer the following questions to determine your Emotional Type. Then read the short profile about a woman who fits the profile.

The Revved Up and Anxious Type

Do you experience one or more of the following symptoms?

	YES	NO
Feeling anxious or panicky		
Irritability		
Rage		
Insomnia		
Rapid thoughts		
Feeling overwhelmed		

- If you answered yes to one or more of the symptoms you are the Revved Up and Anxious Type.
- It's likely you have too low a level of the neurotransmitter serotonin and maybe too much norepinephrine. You probably have high GABA levels, which are attempting to calm you down.
- If you would like to take a urine test to determine your exact levels see the Resources for Sanity on page 213.

Meet Lucy:
The Revved Up and Anxious Type

"I had a lot of stress in my life lately. Initially, it seemed like I was able to deal with it, but four weeks ago I started feeling very panicky as if I had adrenalin rushing through my body. Since then, I've had trouble falling asleep at night, and I wake up frequently with a pounding heart, sweats, ringing in my ears, and a brain that will not shut down.

My thoughts are like a movie in fast forward. I worry about everything; I have no appetite and have lost a total of fifteen pounds in four weeks. I really feel like I am going crazy.

"Two weeks ago I called my gynecologist who immediately referred me to a psychiatrist. I was diagnosed with anxiety and given Xanax. Within a few days of starting the medication, I started feeling odd, disconnected, and not really like myself. I am still getting less than four hours of sleep per night, and during the day I am constantly wondering why I feel the way I do. I am stuck in an obsessive loop; and my friends, family members, and coworkers are sick of listening to me. Really, I talk to anyone I can and go on-line many times a day in a desperate search to find out what is really wrong with me.

Everyone, regardless of her Emotional Type, should follow Mia's Basic Supplement Plan on page 121. The recommendations are also listed on Your Emotional Rescue Plan worksheet. Learn more about all the supplements in Step Three.

"Everyone gives me a different recommendation for something to read, listen to, take, or do. My pantry has become a pharmacy where I store at least fifty bottles of over-the-counter vitamins, along with herbs and soy supplements, but nothing helps me find any comfort. I have seen a Chinese herbalist, acupuncturist, and chiropractor, and my bank account is in serious trouble. Sometimes my symptoms get better for about half a day, but then I turn around, and I'm lost in the same emotional tailspin. I am completely overwhelmed and exhausted. So here I am, at wit's end. If you can't help me I don't know what I'll do."

Obviously Lucy is anxious, big time. She must raise her serotonin level, which in turn will lower her norepinephrine level if it is high. If you are The Revved Up and Anxious Type this is your plan as well. Copy it into Step Two on your Emotional Rescue Treatment Plan.

The Revved Up and Anxious Emotional Type Supplement Plan

Take these supplements in addition to Mia's Basic Supplement Plan.

Supplement	Dose	Frequency	With food?
5–HTP	50–100 mg	1–2 at bedtime	No

In addition, if your mind is racing, you can't fall a sleep at night, or are very anxious try:

L-theanine Will help if your mind is racing during the day or when waking up at night.	200 mg	1–3 times daily	No
GABA Start if still anxious after few days on 5 HTP	500–1000 mg	1–3 times daily	No

The I Can't Get Off The Couch Type

Refer to your Monthly Symptom Tracker and check off the symptoms that apply.

	YES	NO
Lack of motivation		
Feeling depressed		
Feeling "flat"		
Crying spells		
Feeling withdrawn		
Lack of alertness		

- If you answered YES to having one or more of the symptoms, you are the I Can't Get Off The Couch Type.
- You might experience these symptoms throughout the month or

just one or two weeks before your period. Often women develop these symptoms after menopause when their estrogen level has dropped.

• It's likely you have low levels of the neurotransmitters dopamine and/or norepinephrine with normal levels of GABA.

Meet Maureen:
The I Can't Get Off The Couch Type

"My life has turned into cardboard. Everything looks and tastes like cardboard, and I feel flat. I have a lump of sadness sitting in my throat. I look out the window and the world looks black and white when it used to be in color. My brain feels like a cotton ball. I can't focus on anything I need to do. I used to accomplish one task after the other, but now I am just moving papers and bills around into different piles and not getting anywhere. Things that used to be manageable look daunting. I have absolutely no interest in sex, and my husband is losing patience. I am so overwhelmed; I can't seem to get motivated to do much of anything. I could just sleep all day. I don't care, and sadly somehow I don't care that I don't care."

Mia's Mantra

It is just your chemistry

Maureen feels flat and numb. She needs to raise her levels of dopamine and/or raise her levels of norepinephrine. Conveniently, both can be raised with the same supplements. If you are the Can't get Off the Couch Type this is your plan as well. Copy the plan into Step Two on your worksheet.

The I Can't Get Off The Couch Emotional Type Supplement Plan

Take these supplements in addition to Mia's Basic Supplement. Plan.

Supplement	Dose	Frequency	With food?
L-phenylalanine (free form)	250–500 mg	1–2 in AM	No
L-tyrosine (free form)	250–500 mg	1–2 in AM	No

Meet Susan: The Combination Type

"I could not believe the words *I am so depressed* echoed in my own head—until now. I was always an optimistic woman. My overwhelming sense of sadness, lack of ambition, and sheer frustration freaked me out too. I was laid off for the first time in my life at the age of fifty-six. I knew it wasn't because I wasn't good at the job; in fact I was great at it. Still I'd hear words like, *why bother?* and *what's the point* creeping into my thoughts three, four, even five times a day. I was upset and angry with everyone in sight. I wanted to punch someone, yell at my poor husband, or at least get into an intense argument. I was near tears much of the time and feeling despondent and a little hopeless. My husband didn't much like the woman I had become. He had asked when the 'old me' was coming back and I said, "Maybe never! I have put up with you for thirty-five years, now you are going to have to put up with me!" Fortunately, thanks to rebalancing my brain chemistry, the old Susan is now back, and my husband is still here too."

The Combination Type

Refer to your Monthly Symptom Tracker and check off those symptoms that apply.

SYMPTOMS GROUP ONE

	YES	NO
Feeling anxious or panicky		
Irritability		
Rage		
Insomnia		
Rapid thoughts		
Feeling overwhelmed		

SYMPTOMS GROUP TWO

	YES	NO
Lack of motivation		
Feeling depressed		
Feeling "flat"		
Crying spells		
Feeling withdrawn		
Lack of alertness		

If you answered YES to having one or more of the symptoms in *both* Group One and Group Two, you are The Combination Type.

- You likely have low serotonin and low dopamine and/or norepinephrine with either high or low levels of GABA.

The Combination Type has a spectrum of symptoms from both the Revved Up and Anxious Type and the I Can't Get Off The Couch Type. As an example: you can be experience both irritability and rage while at the same time you feel depressed and withdrawn.

Your Emotional Rescue Plan for the Combination Type involves a two-part process:

- First, you need to calm yourself down.
- Then you will "push the gas pedal" to become more alert and motivated.

Part One: Calming Formula

- Take the supplements listed below. These supplements are the same ones recommended for the the Revved Up and Anxious Type. Taking them will increase your serotonin levels and help calm you down. Take these supplements in addition to Mia's Basic Supplement Plan.

Supplement	Dose	Frequency	With food?
5-HTP	50–100 mg	1–2 at bedtime	No
If your mind is racing, you can't sleep at night, or are anxious try:			
L-theanine Will help if your mind is racing during the day or when waking up at night.	200 mg	1–3 times daily	No
GABA Start if still anxious after few days on 5-HTP.	500–1000 mg	1–3 times daily	No

- Once you start feeling more at peace, your sleep should improve. When you get better sleep, your motivation and focus will improve. For some, motivation, cognition, and focus might not improve until you use the recipe for the I Can't Get Off The Couch Type to increase your levels of dopamine and norepinephrine.
- However, don't do it just yet! If you try to pump up your norepinephrine and dopamine too fast you will experience more anxiety and agitation.
- Stay on the recommended program for the Revved up and Anxious Type two to four weeks. Once you feel less anxious and agitated and you sleep better, you are ready for Part Two, which will increase norepinephrine and dopamine levels.

Part Two: Alertness and Motivation Formula

- In addition to the Revved Up and Anxious Type calming formula and Mia's Basic Supplement Plan, incorporate the protocol recommended for the I Can't Get off the Couch Type listed below. Yes, you will be taking many supplements but it will be worth it. I promise.

Supplement	Dose	Frequency	With food?
*L-phenylalanine (free-form)	250–500 mg	1–2 in AM	No
L-tyrosine (free-form)	250–500 mg	1–2 in AM	No

*Avoid if you have a history of high blood pressure or melanoma.

- Stay on this combination program for four to eight weeks. Watch your mood, alertness, and motivation improve as the supplements L-phenylalanine and L-tyrosine wake up your brain.

Troubleshooting for All of the Emotional Types

If you experience any of the following symptoms after starting the supplements, try making the recommended adjustments.

If you experience:	What to adjust
Anxiety, irritability, agitation, insomnia, panic attacks.	Increase the amount of 5-HTP by 50–100 mg or reduce the amount of L-tyrosine and L-phenylalanine until the anxiety has subsided.
You start feeling flat after taking 5-HTP for several weeks.	Cut back on the amount of the 5-HTP.
You feel drugged and tired while you are taking the GABA.	You are taking too much of GABA. Cut back on the amount of GABA that you are taking.
You feel wired at night and can't fall asleep since you started on the 5-HTP.	Some people cannot take the 5-HTP at night. They get revved up from it. Take the 5-HTP in the early afternoon instead.
You are having really vivid dreams or nightmares.	Take the 5-HTP in the morning or afternoon instead.
You start feeling increasingly tired or fatigue.	Cut back on the amount of GABA or 5-HTP you are taking.
You have been on the 5-HTP and/or GABA for 1–2 weeks and still can't fall asleep.	Take 5-HTP in the afternoon instead of evening (while most people sleep better on 5-HTP, some get jacked up). Increase the GABA to 1000 mg bedtime.
Still wake up during the night.	Increase 5-HTP to 200 mg at bedtime Take 200 mg L-theanine at bedtime.
You have been on the 5-HTP and/or GABA for 1–2 weeks and still feel anxious.	Increase the 5-HTP to 100 mg. in AM and 200 mg at bedtime. Take L-theanine 200 mg.three times a day. Take GABA 500 mg three times a day.

Test Your Neurotransmitter Levels

In my practice I frequently recommend neurotransmitter testing, and I have found urine tests to be most accurate and consistent with my patient's symptoms. Your health care practitioner can order test kits from Neuroscience Inc, (www.neurorelief.com), or Sanesco, (www.sanesco.net). It is a simple urine test done at home and then mailed directly to the lab. The results will be sent to your health care practitioner. The cost of these tests varies from $125–$250 depending on the number of neurotransmitters tested.

Need More Support?

• Go to www.femalebraingoneinsane.com

You will find blogs and chat rooms where you can meet other women coming back to balance and sanity.

Step Three: Food and Supplements to the Rescue

THIS BOOK IS ABOUT ELIMINATING your emotional symptoms due to hormone and brain chemistry imbalances so you can live a happy and thriving life. Although it is not a diet or nutrition bible, I will provide you with the nutrition information you need to keep your biochemistry in optimum function.

I'm sure you, like so many of my curious and intelligent patients, have taken the leap into the baffling and overwhelming world of supplements and tinctures. Women walk into my office for their visits with gigantic shopping bags, filled to the brim with a cornucopia of pills, creams, sprays, and lozenges. Their kitchen cabinets and pantries have no more room for food! They have built their own mini-pharmacies filled with everything under the sun.

They have tried every kind of magic solution for female troubles from every source. The Internet suggests a myriad of panaceas, and even if you are a skeptic, you might find yourself purchasing the promise of health from the elixir of bee pollen to various soy extracts. The truth is, many sites give contradictory information or worse, poorly

As you read this chapter, make sure you have Your Emotional Rescue Plan worksheet and pen in hand. This step teaches you about the benefits of supplementation and good nutrition. You'll also learn everything you need to know to commit to a better diet, one that feeds your brain what it needs to be healthy and content. Make sure to fill in the foods you will eat and those you will avoid on Your Emotional Rescue Plan worksheet.

researched data on what to do and what to take to find your way back to health. The twenty-one-year-old earthmama's daughter at the health food store may have become your go-to resource for guidance.

Most salespeople who work in vitamin and supplement stores do not have the education required to make sound recommendations to improve your brain chemistry and your hormonal balance. Cocktails of black cohosh, St. John's wort, and a homeopathic rescue remedy, or a potentially toxic phytoestrogen can leave your wallet empty and your health worse off than ever. Some herb and supplement combinations can actually interfere with your hormonal function by blocking the estrogen receptors. What a waste of time, money, and hope when you may end up more imbalanced than you were in the first place.

How do you know that what you take is what you need to feel better? How do you know if the products you buy are super potent, contaminated, or even contain anything remotely connected to what is listed on the label that is next to impossible to read? Is the company you buy products from testing their supplements to verify quality and purity to insure that they are free from pesticides, bacteria, and heavy metals? So many raw materials in herbs and supplements come from China and India, where sanitation and quality practices are not what we expect. Beware, many U.S. manufacturing companies source out the cheapest raw materials possible, and the vast majority do little or no testing of their source materials or of their finished products. Yes, they create an affordable vitamin. But do you want to swallow it?

How do you research everything you put in your mouth, especially when you are compromised emotionally and physically? After years of research and keeping current with the latest studies and journal entries plus over twenty years of clinical practice, I feel confident sharing my knowledge and experience about supplements with you.

My aim is to modify your biochemistry so that you feel emotionally balanced and happy again. That's a tall order, but it is something I do every day. Therefore, rest assured, the specific brand names I recommend on my website are produced by companies that assure product quality and purity. Moreover, the dosage amounts I recommend are the least amount of product necessary to achieve the best result possible.

This chapter addresses:

- The types of nutrients you need to keep your brain happy.
- Why you need to take nutritional supplements.
- What amino acids are and how they balance your brain chemistry.
- Foods to enjoy.
- Foods you should avoid.

Your Amazing Brain

Your brain is an amazing organ. It is extremely adaptive and will do everything it can to keep you emotionally balanced for as long as possible. The brain is not something fixed in concrete but rather an ever-changing, learning entity. It is as malleable as a lump of wet clay and has the ability to rewire itself, not only in infancy, as scientists have long known, but also into old age. This phenomenon is called neuroplasticity. For neuroplasticity to occur, the brain needs the proper food and nutrients. Just like your car needs the right fuel to run efficiently, your brain needs the right nutrients, or it will malfunction. Without the right fuel or nutrition, your brain function slowly deteriorates, you feel like you are melting down, and chronic anxiety, depression, fatigue, insomnia, memory loss, and difficulty focusing can govern your daily life.

Although your brain represents only about two percent of your body weight, it uses more than 20 percent of all your energy—consuming half of the blood sugar circulating in your bloodstream, one-fourth of your nutrients, and one-fifth of all the oxygen you inhale. Even in the best of times your brain can become malnourished. A malfunctioning brain expresses itself with symptoms reflected in your emotions, moods, thoughts, and behaviors. These symptoms tell you something is out of whack.

Therefore, your brain needs fuel from the right nutritional sources to keep it functional, alive, and well. Fortunately, when it is fed properly, your brain responds quickly. With a well-nourished brain, you feel vibrant and happy, and only then will you be able to make the right decisions about work, finances, relationships, and life issues.

Ninety-two percent of us are deficient in one or more of the essential vitamins and minerals, and more than ninety-nine percent of us are deficient in the essential fatty acids. Dieting or poor nutrition malnourish the brain and contribute to these deficiencies—and we end up lacking amino acids, essential vitamins, minerals, and fats. These deficiencies cause a shortage in the creation and circulation of neurotransmitters causing emotional discomfort and cravings for certain foods—most often carbohydrates like sugar and alcohol. For example, a shortage of the neurotransmitter dopamine reduces feelings of pleasure and motivation, while a lack of GABA produces feelings of restlessness, tension, and anxiety.

Amino Acid Therapy

In Chapter 1 you learned about your brain chemistry and the important function of your neurotransmitters including dopamine, serotonin, GABA, and norepinephrine. Brain chemistry cannot exist without amino acids. Amino acids are the building blocks of protein, and amino acids create your brain chemistry. A total of twenty amino acids are required to create your brain chemistry; but only eleven are manufactured by the body. You can only get the other nine through the foods you eat and the supplements you take. Research shows that when the brain has adequate supplies of amino acids (the building blocks, think Lego) for brain chemicals, emotional behavior tends to be normal. You feel good. Inadequate or imbalanced supplies of amino acids lead to deficits or imbalances in neurotransmitters, causing emotional meltdowns and uncontrolled behavior.

Unfortunately, it is nearly impossible to attain the ideal brain chemistry for optimum health through food alone. A healthy diet certainly helps. You can eat bananas and drink milk to increase tryptophan or serotonin. You can enjoy eggs and other proteins such as cheese to increase phenylalanine, which contributes to the production of dopamine. It's a great habit to eat well, but no matter how well you eat, you will not have a sufficient production of the neurotransmitters you need to keep your brain fed and happy.

Amino acid therapy is the best way to positively influence and improve your brain chemistry. When you take supplemental amino acids to help build and then balance neurotransmitters, you are directly affecting your brain's health.

Six Key Amino Acids

Although twenty amino acids help build brain chemistry, six of them are particularly important for the female brain. Make sure to take the amino acids I recommended for your emotional type as outlined in Step Two.

5-Hydroxytryptophan (5-HTP)

5-HTP is a compound produced in the body from the amino acid called tryptophan. Brain cells synthesize 5-HTP in a two-step process that begins with tryptophan, which comes from dietary sources such as turkey and milk. Once absorbed into the cell, tryptophan is converted into 5-HTP, the precursor to the neurotransmitter serotonin (for peace and calming) and the hormone melatonin, which helps in sleep regulation.

There are several advantages for taking 5-HTP, as compared to L-tryptophan, to elevate brain serotonin levels. The main one is simple: 5-HTP is one-step closer to metabolically building serotonin than tryptophan. In other words, 5-HTP more readily converts to serotonin than tryptophan does. Tryptophan turns into 5-HTP, which turns into serotonin. Unlike tryptophan, 5-HTP is not produced by bacterial fermentation or chemical synthesis. It is extracted from the seeds of the Griffonia plant.

Tyrosine

Tyrosine supports thyroid function and is a precursor to dopamine and norepinephrine, both strong antidepressants as well as excitants. Do not take tyrosine if you suffer from anxiety or panic attacks. Tyrosine is made from the amino acid phenylalanine. Vitamins B$_6$, C, iron, magnesium, copper, manganese, and zinc work with tyrosine to metabolize it into norepinephrine and dopamine. Take tyrosine in the morning to prevent interference with sleep.

L-phenylalanine

L-phenylalanine is an essential amino acid—meaning the body does not make it—it must be ingested. Inside the body, phenylalanine converts into tyrosine. Tyrosine then produces the neurotransmitters dopamine and norepinephrine, which supports thyroid production. L-phenylalanine has been shown to elevate mood, increase physical and mental energy, sex drive, and motivation. L-phenylalanine also helps to suppress your appetite and can assist in maintaining a healthy weight. Symptoms of L-phenylalanine deficiency include confusion, lack of energy, decreased alertness, decreased memory, and diminished appetite. Avoid L-phenylalanine if you have a history of hyperthyroidism, hypertension, anxiety, or melanoma.

Mia's Mantra
You are safe

L-theanine

L-theanine is the predominant amino acid in green tea leaves. Research shows that L-theanine can create a sense of relaxation approximately thirty minutes after ingestion. It works by directly stimulating the production of alpha brain waves, creating a state of deep relaxation and mental alertness similar to what is achieved through meditation. In addition, L-theanine helps with the formation of the inhibitory neurotransmitter GABA. L-theanine is a wonderful amino acid because it calms you down without sedating you in the process.

L-taurine

L-taurine is an amino acid that has a calming and antianxiety effect on the brain. L-taurine counters the "up" effects of dopamine and norepinephrine by helping to stabilize the excitability of the membranes in the nervous system. It is both a neuroinhibitor and a neurotransmitter.

GABA

GABA is an amino acid that is in itself a neurotransmitter. It has a calming effect on the brain as it inhibits the excitatory neurotransmitters dopamine and norepinephrine. Tranquilizers such as Valium and Xanax work by increasing the effectiveness of GABA.

Supplements for Optimum Health

My basic nutritional supplement plan can benefit women of all ages (from teenagers to seniors) regardless of their symptoms, emotional type, or hormonal phase. Women need these basic supplements to maintain good health because the food we consume today does not give us all the vitamins, minerals, and essential fatty acids required to maintain a healthy female brain. Mia's Basic Supplement Plan will serve as a foundation for everyone regardless of Emotional Type. The recommendations for the emotional types *will not* work effectively without the Basic Supplement Plan. Remember, vitamins and minerals are the cofactors or coenzymes that make virtually every biochemical process in your body function, so without them your mood and behavior may be affected. Taking these supplements should be a regular part of your daily regimen and will support your natural biochemistry leading to optimal health. You should take these supplements in addition to those recommended for your hormonal phase and emotional type.

Mia's Basic Supplement Plan

Nutritional Supplement	Total Daily Amount
A high-potency multivitamin and mineral formula	Determined by brand. See my recommend-starting on page 123.

Take the following vitamins in addition to the multivitamin to reach daily total amounts indicated below.

Vitamin B_{12}	1000–2000 mcg
Folic Acid	800 mcg
Vitamin B_6	50–100 mg
EPA Omega-3 DHA Omega-3	600 mg 400 mg
Calcium (elemental)	500–800 mg
Magnesium	400–600 mg
Vitamin D_3	2000–3000 IU
Probiotics	10–20 billion organisms

Note: For specific recommendations on brands and dosages please visit www.femalebrain goneinsane.com. The nutritional supplements recommended on my website are professional grade products. They are manufactured by companies that have completed all the steps required to ensure high standards of quality and purity.

Multivitamins

Multivitamins contain micronutrients like vitamins, minerals, and trace elements along with other nutrients essential for healthy brain function. Vitamin deficiency can have an adverse affect on brain function. A good multivitamin should contain all the B vitamins that I recommend. The B vitamins are essential to mental and emotional well-being. They cannot be stored in our bodies, so we depend entirely on our daily diet to supply them. B vitamins are destroyed by alcohol, birth control pills, refined sugars, nicotine, and caffeine, so it is no surprise that many people may be deficient in them.

- Vitamin B_1 (thiamine): The brain uses this vitamin to help convert glucose, or blood sugar, into fuel. Without it, the brain rapidly runs out of energy, which can lead to fatigue, depression, irritability, anxiety, and even thoughts of suicide.
- Vitamin B_3 (niacin): Deficiencies of vitamin B_3 can produce agitation and anxiety, as well as mental and physical slowness.
- Vitamin B_5 (pantothenic acid): Symptoms of deficiency are fatigue, chronic stress, and depression. Vitamin B_5 is needed for hormone formation and the uptake of amino acids and the brain chemical acetylcholine, which combine to prevent certain types of depression.
- Vitamin B_6 (pyridoxine): This vitamin aids in the processing of amino acids, which are the building blocks of all proteins and some hormones. It is needed in the manufacture of serotonin, melatonin and dopamine.
- Vitamin B_{12}: Deficiency in vitamin B_{12} can cause mood swings, paranoia, irritability, confusion, dementia, hallucinations, or mania, eventually followed by appetite loss, dizziness, weakness, shortage of breath, heart palpitations, diarrhea, and tingling sensations in the extremities. Deficiencies take a long time to develop, since the body stores a three- to five-year supply in the liver. When shortages do occur, they are often due to a lack of intrinsic factor, an enzyme that allows vitamin B_{12} to be absorbed in the intestinal tract. Since intrinsic factor diminishes with age, older people are more prone to B_{12} deficiencies.

- Folic acid: Folic acid has been proven to provide support for healthy nervous system function and a healthy mood. Poor dietary habits contribute to folic acid deficiencies, as do illness, alcoholism, and various drugs, including aspirin, birth control pills, barbiturates, and anticonvulsants. Folic acid is usually administered along with vitamin B_{12}, since a B_{12} deficiency can mask a folic acid deficiency.

    Folic acid deficiency may increase the risk of depression. Antidepressants tend to work better when taken with folic acid. The preferred form of folic acid is 5-methyltetrahydrofolate (5-MTHF) a highly bioavailable form of folate easily absorbed and readily usable by cells. This is the only form of folate that can cross the blood-brain barrier. It requires no additional metabolic steps to be used by the body.

- The antioxidants: The antioxidants (the body's ever-vigilant army that searches out and destroys free radicals) in multivitamins such as vitamin C, vitamin E, and beta-carotene, help protect brain cells from free-radical damage (cell destruction) caused by environmental pollution and toxins. Also, vitamin C is needed for tyrosine to be converted to dopamine and norepinephrine.

- Iron: Many multivitamins contain iron. You will only need iron in your multivitamin if you are still menstruating. Supplementing with iron when you are no longer menstruating can lead to abnormally high levels of iron increasing the risk of cardiovascular disease and stroke.

The multivitamin-mineral you choose to take should contain the following:

Vitamin A..1000–3000 IU
Vitamin C..500–1000 mg

Vitamin D ....500–800 IU

Vitamin E as mixed tocopherols ....400 IU

Vitamin B$_1$ (thiamine)...25–50 mg

Vitamin B$_2$ (riboflavin) ....25–50 mg

Vitamin B$_3$ (Niacinamide) ....30–100 mg

B$_6$ (Pyrodoxine) ....25–50 mg

Folic Acid (ideally as mixed folic acids including

    methyl-folate) ....800 mcg

Vitamin B$_{12}$ (ideally as methylcobalamin)....................500–1000 mcg

Biotin..150–500 mcg

Panthothenic Acid ....50–500 mg

Iodine ....25–75 mcg

Zinc...10–30 mg

Copper...1–2 mg

Selenium..100–200 mcg

Manganese ....3–5 mg

Chromium ....100–400 mcg

Molybdenum ....25–100 mcg

Boron...1–2 mg

Alpha Lipoic Acid ....20–100 mg

Iron (only for menstruating women) ....12–18 mg

Omega-3 Fatty Acids

Over the last decade, neuroscientists have found that essential fatty acids such as eicosapentaenoic acid (EPA) and docosahexaenoic acid (DHA) are crucial to the very structure of the brain. *Essential* means you must get these EFAs from the food you eat. Your body cannot manufacture them. Too little DHA concentrations in brain cell membranes correlate to a decline in structural and functional integrity of the tissue.

Several recent studies have confirmed that the lack of DHA also increases your vulnerability to depression.

Although these essential fatty acids are necessary to support healthy brain structure and function, they are shockingly scarce in the typical American diet. Research indicates that when America went on its low-fat diet craze about 25 years ago, we threw out all dietary fats, including beneficial omega-3 fatty acids like EPA and DHA causing an ever-increasing caseload of people with depression.

Most omega-3 fatty acid supplements are made from fish oil. Because fish oil can thin the blood, individuals who use blood-thinning medications such as Coumadin or who have increased bleeding tendencies should consult a physician before using fish oil. Make sure you get your fish oil from a company that certifies purity from the contamination of heavy metals and pesticides.

Calcium

The body contains more calcium than any other mineral. Ninety to ninety-nine percent of the calcium in the body forms bone tissue. The other five percent plays a critical role in nervous system function and muscle contractions

Susan Thys-Jacobs, an endocrinologist at St. Luke-Roosevelt Hospitals, found that calcium supplementation could relieve the physical and emotional toll of PMS by almost 50 percent. At least half of the 497 women she studied who supplemented with calcium experienced fewer mood swings, less depression or sadness, anxiety or nervousness; breast tenderness, bloating and other aches and pains.

When purchasing calcium supplements, look for the *elemental calcium* content, not the total content. For instance, a pill containing 500 mg of calcium carbonate provides 200 mg of elemental calcium.

Hence, one pill in this example only provides 200 mg of calcium, not 500 mg. I usually recommend calcium citrate or calcium carbonate for best absorption with the daily dose of elemental calcium of 500 to 800 mg.

Magnesium

Magnesium, often referred to as the "anti-stress" mineral, has a calming action, it relaxes nerves and muscles and reduces the effects of stress. A deficiency of magnesium causes many symptoms usually associated with PMS, such as irritability, depression, confusion, and muscle aches. Depressed patients tend to have low magnesium levels. Magnesium seems to help improve premenstrual mood changes. Magnesium glycinate is a well-absorbed form, with minimum laxative effects. I usually recommend 400–600 mg daily. More is sometimes needed for patients suffering from migraines.

Vitamin D₃

Vitamin D₃ is the physiologically active form of Vitamin D, also known as calcitriol. Vitamin D₃ helps the brain produce serotonin, a neurotransmitter critical to emotional health. Vitamin D₃ deficiency can contribute to negative emotions such as depression. Likewise, increased vitamin D consumption elevates mood and promotes a positive outlook.

Vitamin D is known as the hormone of sunlight. Supplementation with vitamin D may prevent seasonal depression. Exposure to sunlight enables the skin to produce vitamin D. As the days grow shorter and colder in winter, the body may be unable to produce adequate amounts of vitamin D. Individuals living in colder climates where the daylight hours shorten significantly at risk for vitamin D deficiency and the resulting winter blues. The latest research shows that vitamin D3 defi-ciency is linked to a surprising number of other health conditions such as, back pain, cancer, both insulin resistance and pre-eclampsia during pregnancy, impaired immunity and macular degeneration. I recom-mend a daily dose of 2000–3000 IU of vitamin D3.

Probiotics: The Healthy Bacteria

Not only are we what we eat, but we are also comprised of what we absorb. To optimally break down and absorb nutrients in the digestive tract, we need to have adequate amounts of probiotics, which are known as the healthy bacteria. A healthy digestive track is home to lit-erally trillions of individual bacteria and more than 500 different species of microflora. The good bacteria, or probiotics, in our intes-tines support overall health, natural immunity, and healthy digestion. The two most prevalent probiotics are *Lactobacilli,* which make up the majority of probiotics living in the small intestine, and *Bifidobacteria,* the most prevalent beneficial probiotic living in the large intestine. Most healthy people have 100 times more *Bifidobacteria* than *Lactobacilli.*

Science has shown that as we age, the number of healthy bacteria in our digestive tract begins to decline. As a result, older adults have a greater risk of suffering from digestive conditions such as constipation, diarrhea, and irritable bowel syndrome (IBS), as well as a decrease in overall immune function. *Bifidobacteria* in particular begin to decline considerably around age 50, so choosing a daily maintenance probiotic with a high *Bifidobacteria* count is recommended for older adults.

There are a few important points to consider when choosing the ideal probiotic formula. For seniors, look for an effective multistrain formula with high levels of *Bifidobacteria* for maximum support. Enteric-coated capsules are also important, as they help protect the beneficial bacteria from the acidic environment of the stomach and deliver them directly to the intestines where they're needed most. To find out your specific need for beneficial bacteria, your health care practitioner can order stool tests that will tell you your balance of friendly bacteria. I use Genova Diagnostics and Metamerix (see page 212) to evaluate my patients gut health. For recommendations of specific manufacturers and products, visit www.femalebraingoneinsane.com

Food for Your Brain

We all know it is important to eat a healthy diet. However, did you know that eating certain foods and drinks can actually make you happier? Recent studies show that nutrients play a significant role in maximizing your brain's potential, so what you eat can affect brain function and your mood.

Foods contain six basic nutritional components: proteins, carbohydrates, fats, vitamins, minerals, and water. Without a sufficient supply of all six, the human brain will rapidly fail to thrive or function. Some foods are rich with nutrients, while others are nutritionally bankrupt. As you become more nutritionally conscious and pay attention to what you eat, you will certainly help to keep your brain working at its best.

I recommend my patients start the day with a protein smoothie in addition to eating protein at least two times a day. Mia's Brain-boosting Mind-soothing Protein Smoothie is an easy and delicious way to start your day with a nutritious beginning and a healthy dose of protein. It is also a good way for vegetarians to ensure adequate protein intake each day.

Protein powder is a key ingredient in the smoothie. Choose rice protein powder if you have food sensitivities, allergies, or intestinal issues.

READER/CUSTOMER CARE SURVEY

HEFG

We care about your opinions! Please take a moment to fill out our online Reader Survey at **http://survey.hcibooks.com.**
As a **"THANK YOU"** you will receive a **VALUABLE INSTANT COUPON** towards future book purchases
as well as a **SPECIAL GIFT** available only online! Or, you may mail this card back to us.

(PLEASE PRINT IN ALL CAPS)

First Name _____ MI. _____ Last Name _____

Address _____ City _____

State _____ Zip _____ Email _____

1. Gender
- ☐ Female ☐ Male

2. Age
- ☐ 8 or younger
- ☐ 9-12   ☐ 13-16
- ☐ 17-20 ☐ 21-30
- ☐ 31+

3. Did you receive this book as a gift?
- ☐ Yes   ☐ No

4. Annual Household Income
- ☐ under $25,000
- ☐ $25,000 - $34,999
- ☐ $35,000 - $49,999
- ☐ $50,000 - $74,999
- ☐ over $75,000

5. What are the ages of the children living in your house?
- ☐ 0 - 14   ☐ 15+

6. Marital Status
- ☐ Single
- ☐ Married
- ☐ Divorced
- ☐ Widowed

7. How did you find out about the book?
(please choose one)
- ☐ Recommendation
- ☐ Store Display
- ☐ Online
- ☐ Catalog/Mailing
- ☐ Interview/Review

8. Where do you usually buy books?
(please choose one)
- ☐ Bookstore
- ☐ Online
- ☐ Book Club/Mail Order
- ☐ Price Club (Sam's Club, Costco's, etc.)
- ☐ Retail Store (Target, Wal-Mart, etc.)

9. What subject do you enjoy reading about the most?
(please choose one)
- ☐ Parenting/Family
- ☐ Relationships
- ☐ Recovery/Addictions
- ☐ Health/Nutrition
- ☐ Christianity
- ☐ Spirituality/Inspiration
- ☐ Business Self-help
- ☐ Women's Issues
- ☐ Sports

10. What attracts you most to a book?
(please choose one)
- ☐ Title
- ☐ Cover Design
- ☐ Author
- ☐ Content

TAPE IN MIDDLE; DO NOT STAPLE

BUSINESS REPLY MAIL
FIRST-CLASS MAIL PERMIT NO 45 DEERFIELD BEACH, FL

POSTAGE WILL BE PAID BY ADDRESSEE

Health Communications, Inc.
3201 SW 15th Street
Deerfield Beach FL 33442-9875

FOLD HERE

Comments

Stay away from whey protein if you are lactose intolerant and soy protein if you are allergic or sensitive to soy. If you are watching your weight, you can reduce the calories in the smoothie by using only half the liquid recommended and diluting the rest with water. To reduce the sugar content even more, omit the juice and add a small amount of stevia, a natural sweetener made from a tropical plant native to South America. Its extract has up to 300 times the sweetness of sugar. Stevia does not raise insulin levels.

Mia's Brain-boosting Mind-soothing Protein Smoothie

I–2 cups orange, apple, or cranberry juice, or yogurt, soy, or almond milk

1 tablespoon flax meal (ground up flax seeds)

20 grams whey protein powder (unless you have food sensitivities to dairy then replace the whey protein with soy or rice protein)

½–1 cup frozen berries (blueberries, raspberries, strawberries), organic preferred

Process in a blender and drink right away.

Note: If you experience gas or bloating try using less of the flax meal.

Even in the best of times your brain is often malnourished from not getting enough protein, which is then reflected in your emotions and behavior. Amino acids that come from the protein you eat are the building blocks of your brain's network of neurotranmitters. Your body breaks down dietary protein into the amino acids it uses to assemble the 50,000 different proteins it needs to function—including neurotransmitters and chromosomes, hormones, and enzymes. Fortunately, your brain quickly benefits from proper nutrition—even from a single meal. Great sources of protein are organic meats, cheese, eggs, fish, poultry, and game.

Carbohydrates Fuel the Brain

While the brain's primary energy fuel is glucose, the brain cannot store it. Therefore, once carbohydrates are broken down into glucose by the body, the glucose is then carried to the brain by the bloodstream where it is used immediately as energy by nerve cells. The brain uses about 60 percent of the glucose you eat. The brain uses glucose to perform many functions including thinking, short-term and long-term memory, and sleeping.

According to the Institute of Medicine, the brain needs at least 130 grams of carbohydrates per day in order to function properly. Most low-carb diets recommend less than that even though the latest research shows that eating a diet too low in carbohydrates negatively influences brain functioning.

Carbohydrates enhance the absorption of tryptophan, which is converted into serotonin in the brain. Within about thirty minutes of eating a carbohydrate meal you will feel more calm and relaxed. The effects will last several hours.

It is important to avoid simple carbohydrates often found in junk food because the glucose gives the brain a short-lived sugar high, often followed by a crash that makes you feel hungry, dizzy, and tired. Complex carbohydrates, on the other hand, are packed with fiber, vitamins, and minerals that supply the brain with a steady stream of glucose, which enhances brain function.

Examples of complex carbohydrates are whole grains, fruits, beans, and vegetables. Honey, corn syrup, table sugar, fruit juice, milk, yogurt, molasses, maple syrup, and brown sugar are examples of the simple carbohydrates you should avoid.

Fats Build Your Brain

No offense, but you have a fat head! About two-thirds of your brain is composed of fats, but not just any type of fat. Your brain is composed of essential fatty acids (EFAs), and for optimal brain function, you need to incorporate essential fatty acids in your diet.

Fats determine how many nerve cells you will have available for intelligence, learning, memory, attention, concentration, and mood. Fat molecules help determine how much of which type of neurotransmitters your brain cells will make and release. Unless you get the right kinds of fats in the right amounts, your brain tissue may become starved. When this happens, the outer membranes of your brain cells stiffen and shrivel. The rich chemical flood of neurotransmitters may dry up or become short-circuited, so they are unable to gain entry to neurons and carry messages from neuron to neuron.

Eating healthy fats, known as EFAs, as part of a balanced diet improve the health of the skin, brain function, and cell membranes. Choose from nuts, nut butters, olives, avocados, coconut oil, butter, extra virgin olive oil (omega-6), and flaxseed oil (omega-3). Flaxseed oil is highly unstable, and it must be kept refrigerated in an enclosed container so that it is not exposed to oxygen and light. Other healthy oils include fish, palm, coconut, and sesame oils.

Cold-water fish such as salmon, trout, sardines, arctic char, mackerel, herring, and sole provide high amounts of EFAs. Other good sources include shark, swordfish, king mackerel, and tilefish—but because these fish may contain high levels of mercury, pregnant women and children should avoid them. Others should only eat these fish once a week.

Mia's Quick Tips for A Happy Brain

- Start your morning with a breakfast high in protein— preferably with Mia's Brain-boosting and Mind-soothing Smoothie.
- Coffee is not a meal . . . even with milk.
- Eat at least three 15–20 gram protein meals a day.
- Don't skip meals.
- Keep your blood sugar balanced.
- Avoid artificial sweeteners, hydrogenated fats, and sugar.
- Limit your alcohol intake.
- Drink eight or more glasses of water a day.
- Read labels. Eliminate packaged and processed foods from your diet. If you can't pronounce something you read on the label, don't put it in your mouth.

Foods That Impair Brain Functioning

With all the wonderful, healthy foods available to you, making smart choices should be easy. However, even some innocent-looking foods (white flour, for example) pose potential problems for your brain chemistry:

- Don't drink alcohol. Although red wine in moderation can reduce the risk of cardiovascular disease, all alcohol is counterproductive when it comes to mood. Acute and chronic alcohol consumption can have both subtle as well as dramatic effects on the brain and how well it functions. For example, damage to the brain can occur through alcohol-induced deficiencies in nutrition, through liver disease, and through alterations of hormones and neurotransmitters. Alcohol has a direct action on the brain as a depressant. If you are depressed, drinking alcohol might initially calm you down but it will make you more depressed over the long haul. Alcohol can cause an imbalance among the neurotransmitters by suppressing the excitatory neurotransmitter glutamate while activating the calming neutransmitter GABA. In the end, you might end up too sedated and depressed, with a lack of motivation and energy.

- Avoid artificial food colorings. When you read food labels, you will see food colors (such as FD&C Blue #1, Red #3) in all sorts of foods such as salmon, baked goods, puddings, granola, juices, fruit snacks cereals, and more. Even the skin on the oh-so-natural orange can be dyed to give it that extra orangey hue. Yes, some companies actually dye food in an effort to make it look more appealing and healthy. However, food coloring is very harmful to your brain. It can change the way you behave, causing hyperactive behavior, focusing difficulties, and lack of impulse control.

  Red food coloring actually contains a chemical called carmine, which is derived from mashed up beetles raised in Peru and the Canary Islands. The mashed beetle bodies are strained to obtain a red liquid. That liquid, made from the insects, is processed into children's food and candy, and that's just for starters. It is also an ingredient in some yogurt to give it that ripe-red, fresh strawberry color.

- Stay away from artificial sweeteners: Aspartame is a commonly used artificial sweetener found in diet sodas and most chewing gums. Aspartame contains chemical toxins that can disrupt your neuro-transmitter functions causing symptoms such as migraines, depression, seizures, attention deficit disorder, angry rages, joint pain, muscle spasm, and it can mimic diseases like multiple sclerosis, chronic fatigue syndrome, and fibromyalgia.

The FDA has had more complaints about aspartame (NutraSweet, Equal, Canderel, Spoonfuls, and DiabetiSweet) than any other food additive, and yet it is still on the Generally Regarded As Safe list despite its strong association with brain tumors and seizures. Splenda is another fake sugar that can adversely affect the body in several ways because it is a chemical substance and not natural sugar. I recommend you wean off sugars—particularly artificial ones—completely, but if you still need to sweeten your food, choose safe sweeteners like raw (unpasteurized) honey, organic maple syrup, or stevia. Stevia cannot be sold as a sweetener in the United States, but as a dietary supplement. The harvested and dried leaves of the herb are extremely sweet, about 300 times sweeter than conventional sugar.

• Watch your sugar intake. Keeping your blood sugar levels in balance is one of the most important things you can do for your health. It truly maximizes your brainpower. Dramatic shifts in blood sugar levels hamper brain focus, your ability to concentrate, and your memory. If you think about it, about an hour after a high-sugar meal you tend to feel tired and struggle with a fuzzy brain. Sugar can raise adrenaline levels, and therefore, can cause anxiety and insomnia. It can also alter your brain waves, which affects your mind's ability to think clearly.

Sugar also affects your hormone levels. A high-sugar diet increases insulin levels, which block the receptors for your hormones. The result? You suffer hormonal deficiency symptoms such as hot flashes, night sweats, and depression.

• Ban hydrogenated fats. During the past century, modern food processing techniques have actually altered the good fats we need for proper brain development and functioning. Scientists created trans-fatty acids, which are chemically altered from hydrogenated liquid oils so that they can withstand food production processes and to provide a longer shelf life. Trans-fatty acids are found in many processed foods including french fries, margarine, potato chips, and crackers. When you eat these foods, the trans-fatty acids replace the healthy fat (DHA) in the brain cell membranes and ultimately impair the communication from one brain cell to another. Trans-fatty acids are rarely found in nature and are mostly manmade.

• Say no to white flour. White flour is made from chemically processed wheat flour, and it takes a lot of processing to turn whole-wheat flour into white flour. The end result is missing the two most nutritious and fiber-rich parts of the wheat: the outside bran layer and the germ. The reason white flour is white and not brown is that it is chemically bleached, just like the whites in your laundry. Therefore, when you are eating white bread, you are also eating residual chemical bleach. Not exactly something your brain needs to thrive.

Now you have learned how to bolster your brainpower through healthy eating. With the addition of these recommendations, you will experience a definite improvement in how you feel—particularly if you suffer from mild or moderate depression, anxiety, or irritability. Embracing healthy eating habits will have a dramatic and revitalizing impact on your mood almost immediately.

Step Four: Stress-buster and Life-improvement Techniques

I AM NOT A LIFESTYLE COACH, nor will I pretend to be one. I am a health practitioner with an expertise in functional medicine. That said, the recommendations I make in this chapter are based on what I have gleaned from my patients as well as lessons I have learned walking through fifty plus years of life on this planet. My experiences have enabled me to develop a very simple and straightforward approach to help you lessen the stress in your life so that you can move forward and create the life you want. Please don't worry. I will not ask you to make any big changes. You've already done so much! So, dear woman, here is the basic game plan to manage you stress.

As you read this chapter, make sure you have Your Emotional Rescue Plan and pen in hand. Step Four gives you the chance to commit to a healthier and less stressful lifestyle. Fill in the appropriate answers and set your goals. You'll feel better for it.

Life is stressful. We can't avoid it. However, too much stress causes all kinds of problems. The good news is, when you have a balanced biochemistry you can endure stress without it wreaking havoc on your system. So please, make sure you follow Your Emotional Rescue Plan and feed yourself the right hormones, supplements, amino acids, and brain foods for optimal balance and protection from the ravages of stress.

Remove Stressors

It's important for you to face what got you into the trenches of imbalance in the first place. Ask yourself, *What are my top five stressors?* Are you struggling with relationships, work, illness, poor nutrition, or too much running around? Once you identify your stressors, you can modify or even eliminate some of what's driving you insane. Pay attention to when you feel a tight gut, a lump in your throat, nervousness, or sweaty palms. What makes you feel uneasy or agitated? Identify your triggers and attempt to cut them out of your life if you can.

I suggest you sit down by yourself or with family members or friends and figure out what seems to stress you out the most. Is it that you are stressed out when you come home from work and everyone is competing for your attention, or is it that your teenager is playing offensive, loud rap music in his room?

You can always ask for a fifteen minute "quite zone" when you come home from work. Find a quiet, peaceful place in the house where you can stretch out alone for fifteen minutes. A little break can make a huge difference on you stress level. You can also ask your teenager to invest in a headset for his loud listening pleasure. Go to Step Four of Your Emotional Rescue Plan worksheet, and list your Top Five Stressors. Now, which ones are you willing and able to tackle?

Change the Way Your Body Responds to Stress

You cannot eliminate every stressor from life; including aging parents, mortgage payments, airborne allergens, and noise. Instead, you can seek help through therapies that will change the way your body responds to these stressors. Let's say you have a really annoying mother-in-law. Every time she calls you, your body reacts with a stress response causing nervousness and anxiety. Maybe she tries to turn your husband against you, manipulates the conversation, and is just too bossy. You can tell yourself, *I won't let this bother me.* You can work with a counselor to sort it all out. After years of experience, I've found therapies such as biofeedback, hypnosis, acupuncture, and neuro-linguistic programming (NLP) will tap into your unconsciousness and actually change the way your nervous system responds to stress, including the kind caused by your mother-in-law.

Before you read another word, take a moment to become aware of yourself. Notice how you are sitting. Are you tense? Are your shoulders glued to your ears? Are you holding your breath? How do you feel right now? Say a word out loud that describes your feeling. Now simply whisper the word "relax" aloud. Then soften your body and slowly inhale and exhale through your nose a few times. Soft, slow. Good.

An excellent NLP therapist works in my office. My patient Juliet had just been through a stressful divorce from an abusive husband, whom she still had to communicate with frequently since they had joint custody of two children. Every time Juliet's husband called, her nervous system flipped into fight or flight causing her to experience serious anxiety attacks and deep fear. Juliet worked with our NLP therapist, and after only a few visits, she no longer reacted the same way. Instead of going into instant panic, her nervous system remained calm. Juliet was able to maintain composure and stay centered.

Neurolingustic programming (NLP) is a general approach to modeling human behavior. It allows you to change, adopt, or eliminate behaviors, as you desire, and gives you the ability to choose your mental, emotional, and physical states of well-being. With NLP, you learn how to grow from every single life experience, thus increasing your ability to create a better quality of life. NLP addresses the mind and language patterns, and it teaches us to change our perceptions and thoughts.

Another useful treatment method called biofeedback uses monitoring devices to help you consciously regulate your bodily functions, such as heart rate, blood pressure, temperature, and anxiety. Seeing your physiology respond to changes in your breathing, for example, is exciting and empowering. Simply put, biofeedback is a means for gaining control of our body processes to increase relaxation, relieve pain, and develop healthier, and more manageable life patterns. Biofeedback is one of several methods approved by the National Institutes of Health (NIH) for use as a complementary therapy for treating chronic pain and insomnia.

Originated in China over 5,000 years ago, acupuncture is based on the belief that living beings have a vital energy, called *qi,* that circulates through twelve invisible energy lines known as meridians on the body. In Chinese medicine, stress, anxiety, depression, or any strong emotion interrupts the smooth flow of *qi* throughout the body. Stress, anger, or any intense emotion acts like a traffic jam, blocking the free flow of energy in the body. For example, often people who are very stressed out complain of upper back, shoulder, and neck pain. This is because stress is causing tension in those areas, blocking the free flow of energy, resulting in pain and tightness. Through acupuncture, these energy blockages can be released. Acupuncturists insert needles into specified points along meridian lines to influence the restore balance to the flow of *qi*. There are more than 1,000 acupuncture points on the body.

Acupuncture also alleviates the symptoms of stress and anxiety by releasing natural pain-killing chemicals in the brain, called endorphins. In addition, acupuncture improves circulation of blood throughout the body, which oxygenates the tissues and cycles out cortisol and waste chemicals. The calming nature of acupuncture also decreases heart rate, lowers blood pressure, and relaxes the muscles.

Hypnosis is a scientifically verified and effective technique used to promote desired changes in your behavior and encourage mental and physical well-being. Our minds work on two levels, conscious and sub-conscious. You think, make decisions, and act mainly with your conscious mind. The subconscious mind, however, is what controls your habits. Hypnosis helps you achieve a deeply relaxed state where your subconscious can focus on and visualize the positive changes you would like to make in your life. Through hypnosis, you become empowered to choose behaviors consciously that will enable you to achieve your goals. Hypnosis has helped many people reduce stress, quit smoking, manage pain, perform better, and accomplish a myriad of other mental and physical tasks. While there are classes and books on the techniques of self-hypnosis, many people use hypnotherapists to achieve the deep state of relaxation and behavioral changes.

Another resource for stress reduction is Healing Rhythms, a personal training tool using state of the art technology with beautiful visuals, soothing sounds, and effective meditation and breathing techniques to help you uncover your body's natural ability to counter the effects of stress. It allows you to witness and transform the rhythms of your mind and body as they play together on the computer screen. You will be able to watch your body respond on screen as you follow the guidance of the world-renowned teachers: Deepak Chopra, Dean Ornish, and Andrew Weil. Each step focuses on a unique and practical meditation, breathing exercise, or guided relaxation to take you closer and closer to your personal goals. Look in the Resources for Sanity section to learn how to find a practitioner in the various modalities.

Most of us are caught up in work, taking care of our families, and striving for material things. Doing and getting seem far more important than simply being. I know better, and I still find it challenging to just rest in the present moment, right now, and allow myself to feel satisfied. The truth is, people who do too much often end up doing too little of what really matters. They spend their lives buzzing from one chore to the next, instead of focusing on the moment and what is really mean-ingful. Most of us fail to take the time to stop and listen to discover what we want or need that will bring us peace and contentment.

Some of us are devoted to keeping a perfectly organized home; others work all of the time and forget what it feels like to play and just spend quality time with friends or family. Our actions create more than just imbalance in our lives. Extreme behaviors can drain us by depleting our immune systems and causing us emotional distress. Sadly, we may end up alienating friends and family, and disliking ourselves as well.

Practice My Antidotes to Stress

Here is a list of antidotes to stress that my patients have found effec-tive. Try practicing as many of them as possible. They will really work to change your life for the better. Most important, as you make these changes don't live your life in isolation. Keep your friends and family as close as possible. Having a circle of women in your life is crucial to give you support, love, honest feedback, perspective, and of course, shared wisdom.

Note five antidotes you will try on Your Emotional Rescue Plan worksheet:

- Take time to breathe
- Love and forgive yourself and others
- Hug a lot
- Stroke a pet
- Laugh
- Pray
- Get counseling
- Listen to a meditation CD
- Take a yoga class
- Try art or music therapy
- Join a community (church, spiritual organizations, parent groups, support groups)
- Lower the bar; stop being a perfectionist
- Sleep more
- Take naps
- Walk in nature
- Cultivate new friends and nurture old ones
- Take time for yourself today, even one minute
- Do less
- Get a massage
- Watch the sunrise or sunset
- Gaze at the horizon
- Take a bath

Cultivate Friendships

Women are not that different from our ancestors 10,000 years ago. Our body and biochemistry and, most important, our stress responses remain the same as the cavewomen of yesteryear who were being chased by tigers and their big hairy husbands. Maybe we stand upright and have stylish shoes now, but we are biochemically designed the same as years ago. Back in the cavewomen days, women washed clothes, made baskets, and collected plants for dinner together. They sat around the fire watching their kids and grandkids, helping each other while talking and listening. They were not in competition with the men, who went off hunting for animals. Nor were they out working fifty-hour weeks, racing through a thousand errands, or living isolated in suburbia.

Today, however, many of us work outside the home to earn a living, we have busy lives, and don't make time for friends. We have lost the sense of support and community we once had with other women. Make an effort to connect with other women, by joining support groups, book clubs, or just take the time to get together with your girlfriends for a weekend away or a nice lunch.

Developing friendships and a sense of belonging is essential to optimal health. Humans are social animals. Your relationships with others greatly influence your mental health, that is: your happiness, self-esteem, and ability to create, love, and work. Several recent studies indicate that women with a solid sense of belonging enjoyed better health than those who felt less connected. Rewarding relationships build self-esteem and fill a void material belongings leave vacant. On an essential level, personal relationships truly improve our health and well-being.

Lower the Bar

You don't need to be perfect. Perfectionism is something that consumes a huge amount of energy while creating stress and anxiety. Lowering the bar does not mean being lazy, sloppy, or slothful. It means realizing that life isn't about perfectionism and that we need to learn to be kind to ourselves and tender-hearted. This is not easy to do. We are competitive and often expected to do everything faster and better. Relentless speed and perfectionism feed stress. Perfectionism stems from holding exceedingly high standards and the need to be in control. We can be perfectionistic in a variety of domains including having high standards for ourselves; feeling pressure from others, such as parents, to act perfectly; and expecting others to be perfect and to meet our high standards.

Sometimes when your emotions feel out of control, your knee-jerk reaction is to grab for something you do have control over. Try to let go of your high expectations and accept life's little imperfections. In your quest to get things "just right" you can often spend excessive amounts of time on a task making small changes when that time could be better spent nurturing your relationships with your children, family, or friends.

Appreciate Life

By now, your biochemistry is well on the road to balance. You have taken charge. It is time to appreciate your inner beauty, time to discover your purpose and your soulful reason for living. This is a wonderful opportunity to grow and explore. Each decade brings us different challenges, lessons, and hopefully, meaning. There are things we would never consider doing at twenty-five that make us feel good and whole at fifty. Each stage of life has a different flavor, rhyme, and reason.

In your thirties and forties your eyes face outward to others. At thirty-five, many of us work so hard at being good moms and wives that it takes all we've got to balance family and jobs to make it all happen. In our forties, we need to be available and strong for our hormonal teenagers, aging parents, and husbands going through their own mid-life sagas, while our own hormones often ride the unpredictable roller coaster of perimenopause. Once in our fifties, we face issues of mortality and aging as well as a new opening to a spiritual part of ourselves we may not have recognized before. Teens move out or go to college. Husbands retire. We may look in the mirror and ask ourselves, *Now what?* or *Who am I?* All of a sudden, your eyes turn inward. Do you even know yourself? Have you ever really been with yourself? What makes you *you*? What do *you* love? What gives *you* pleasure? These questions begin to grow louder as time goes by. The truth is, as you ponder these questions and come up with a few answers along the way, your life will sparkle with a new richness and contentment.

Meet Sally

At forty-five, Sally was riding the hormonal roller coaster of emotions with unpredictable and erratic symptoms characteristic of perimenopause. She sat in my office and began to cry. "Mia, I'm totally out of control. I cannot predict my moods anymore, and I cannot stand how I behave from month to month. My teenage children want to know what is wrong with me. They begged me to seek some help. I feel like a complete failure. And, I worry all the time. What's going to happen when my kids leave home? I stay awake at night and ask myself, *Now what, Sally. What is my purpose?* Before I had children, I was a flight attendant and worked with a great makeup company in Los

Angeles. It was fun back then, but I have no desire to return to that kind of life. I dread the empty nest. How will I fit in? What will I do? I feel totally hopeless and groundless."

I told Sally we needed to adjust her biochemistry, which would change the way she thinks and feels. Then, I turned philosophic. "Sally, please stop feeling so urgent about knowing what's next. Stop swimming upstream to find a solution. It is time to wait and ask. Watch, listen, and see what comes floating down the river of life instead. Ask for guidance and answers, and they will come to you." Sally shared that she was a Christian, and so I suggested she pray. "Please, be still, take the time and listen. Don't run, don't push, don't over exercise. You deserve to breathe, stop the rush, and trust you'll know."

Sally took a deep breath and gently closed her eyes. Then she smiled. "You mean I don't need to figure it out today. Instead I can lie on the couch, put on some music when the kids are off at school and pray?"

"Yes," I said. "That sounds like a good nurturing lifestyle shift."

Remember, there is no need to chase happiness or answers. Try to learn to relax and ask for what you want. Trust me, before you know it, there will be a little sign or clue to show you what to do and what lies ahead.

Take Time to Breathe

Women come to my office every day and tell me their stories. They are often agitated, anxious, or deeply worried. They speak rapidly, spilling their souls in a desperate attempt to be heard. I listen carefully and watch their breathing. Their upper chests move in and out quickly, like little frightened puppies panting after a wild run. These women are wound up, often breathless, and certainly uneasy. Slowly, I explain what is going on with their biochemistry and their female brains and why they feel the way they do.

By the end of the visit they settle down. I see their shoulders drop from their ears. I see their breathing change from upper chest panting to deeper heart or belly breathing. They transform before my eyes by becoming more grounded and at ease. Why? Because someone actually took the time to listen to them. I validate their feelings and symptoms. I assure them that they are not crazy. They trust me, and, in turn, they can finally trust themselves. They have hope. In addition, they have their own Emotional Rescue Plan to take with them when they leave.

It's amazing to experience the power of your own breath—to feel what it's like to inhale deeply and fill the bottom of your lungs with some oxygen. You need oxygen to thrive. I, too, have to watch myself as I shut down my chest and hold my breath even when I am preoccupied with a simple TV show. Why do I forget to breathe? It's an unconscious response, a habit from living in a stressful environment. Moreover, we have all become creatures of the habit of stress.

In yoga and other forms of relaxation and meditation, we learn how to inhale while forming a soft belly that poofs out like a balloon. Called belly breathing, this breath allows you to take in more oxygen then you do when you inhale with regular breathing. Try belly breathing to create a sense of peace.

Sleep More

An old Italian proverb says, "Bed is a medicine." It's true. Lack of sleep increases your stress hormone cortisol and can cause weight gain, mood swings, fatigue, increased irritability, memory loss, and decreased focus, while making it harder for you to fall asleep. Sufficient sleep is essential for daily body repair, rebalance, and rejuvenation. Your cells produce protein molecules while you sleep; and these molecules form the building blocks for your hormones and brain chemistry.

Make your bedroom a sleeping sanctuary. Invest in room-darkening blinds or curtains, and keep the TV and computer away from your sleeping quarters. Your bedroom should be as quiet and as dark as possible to help induce sleep. You need to find a way to love sleep again, so give it the priority it deserves. Of course, you will look and feel better after a good night's sleep and have clearer thoughts, faster reactions, and less fragile emotions. Get those zzzzs back into your life.

Take Naps

A brief, thirty-minute nap benefits heart functioning and hormonal maintenance and helps with brain neuron and cell repair. It also reduces your stress hormones, while it improves alertness, cognition, and memory. Instead of napping, women frequently gulp some coffee or strong tea to keep themselves from nodding off. You may think you are having a bad day when all you need is to curl up somewhere—even outside if it is warm enough—with a cozy blanket to doze off.

In a recent study, researchers at NASA found that a thirty-minute power nap increased cognitive faculties by approximately 40 percent. Another study showed to produce maximum effectiveness the nap must not be too long. If you nap for over forty-five minutes, the beneficial effects seem to disappear, so I suggest you try sticking to a twenty to thirty-five minute power nap.

Maybe you are a staunch anti-napper. Now that you are a little bit older it's time to challenge yourself to stretch the limits. So lie down. Admit it; you might really like it! Find or create a comfortable spot and take a nap. Don't be ashamed! Even five minutes of shut-eye will help you feel refreshed, renewed, and more focused. You'll feel like a new woman.

Happy Napping Tips

- Drop the guilt. You can make those phone calls later.
- Promise yourself one nap every week for starters. Take baby steps.
- An after-lunch siesta makes good sense.
- Try napping different times of the day.
- Put on music. Sip soothing tea. Inhale lavender. Make it a ten-minute ritual.
- Wear clean socks to keep your feet warm.

Make Face-to-Face Time

Our lifestyles have become increasingly dependent on technology—with the growing popularity of online banking, shopping, telecommuting, and personal websites, chat rooms, twitter, and email, it's inevitable we spend less face-to-face time with family and friends. According to a 2007 study of more than 1,000 Americans, 65 percent spend more time with their personal computer than with their spouse. Well, that is not healthy, and long hours in front of the computer increase stress.

Mia's Mantra
You are not going off the deep end

Constantly staring at your computer screen can cause a condition called computer vision syndrome (CVS), which results in neck and back pain, blurred vision, and headaches—symptoms associated with stress. In addition, the constant computer background noise, which is distracting and annoying, contributes to headaches and irritability, two sure signs of stress.

- Don't turn on your computer the moment you wake up.

- Don't check your email every chance you get. Try limiting it to two times a day.
- Do spend more time with friends and family. Try talking in person.

What Makes You Content?

If you had three wishes to create a life of contentment, what would they be? What would your life look and feel like? Who is in it? Where is it? How can you live your life to the fullest? How can you include who and what you truly love? I often ask my patients these questions and encourage them to share their three wishes for contentment. Articulating your dreams will encourage you to stop and actually think about yourself for a moment. Set your goals high and pursue them until they are achieved. As a reminder, record your three wishes for contentment on Your Emotional Rescue Plan.

I usually hear women provide very simple answers. They say they want to spend time away with their girlfriends, lovers, or husbands. They want a change of scenery, a real time-out to unplug from patterns, routines, and computers. They want spa days, massages, and soaks in warm water. What gives you satisfaction?

Foster Intimacy

Intimacy is the experience of being fully who we are in the presence of another who also feels fully who they are. Healthy human beings have a natural need for closeness with others. Intimacy involves both emotional and physical closeness, and is essential for healthy longevity. When we are intimate with another person we can understand and express our true inner being. This gives us meaning and motivation for living happily and joyfully. Intimate relationships are important for managing anxiety and depression.

In the recent past, marriage and family counselors believed that conflict, including arguments, antagonism, and lack of respect for differences, was what eventually led to divorce. However, current research shows that loss of intimacy and affection most likely lead to a broken relationship. While fighting and conflict usually precede a breakup, conflict is the result of a lack of intimacy, not the cause. To protect and preserve your relationship with your significant others, focus on maintaining intimacy and closeness with the important people in your life.

When your hormones change or serotonin levels are low, your sex drive may decrease along with your desire for intimacy. These biochemical changes can cause tension in relationships and marriages. It's important to note: men have sex to feel good; women have sex when they feel good. To feel good, most women want to be appreciated, adored, and cherished. We want to hear how much we are appreciated, adored, and cherished. Yes, we want it in words, not just in actions. Sometimes men fail to recognize our ears are waiting to be seduced before we are.

Make a "Honey-do" List

You have probably heard of the "honey-do" list for such things as a drippy faucet or messy garage. Here are some examples of the "honey-do" list for a sane female brain.

- Listen to me.
- Talk to me.
- Ask me how my day was.

- Tell me you are proud of me.
- Tell me you are a better man or your life is better because of me.
- Make me my favorite cup of tea, and tell me about your day.
- Stroke my forehead, or play with my hair.
- Complement me. Just tell me I look beautiful.
- Bring me fresh flowers. (Please not the ones from the supermarket.)
- Tell me I'm sexy.
- Tell me you want to hold me. Then hold me.
- Thank me for something I did.
- Plan something special—a romantic dinner, a picnic, a weekend away.
- Surprise me.

Create your own "honey-do list" and add it to your Emotional Rescue Plan worksheet. Use examples from this list or make up your own. Give the list to your husband or partner, and ask him to follow through on the suggestions he likes.

Share the Facts

Informing your loved ones about what you have been going through during this difficult time will reinforce your personal connections with them and keep love alive. You have probably acted erratically: distant, scared, and spaced out, unavailable, or any combination of these or other behaviors. Your actions may have created discord between those closest to you. Rebalancing your biochemistry isn't like getting over the flu. It can take a much longer time. Because of our behavior, our loved ones, despite their best intentions, can get angry, impatient, or just fed up. That's all you need while you are trying to get a grip! Many of my patients have asked me how to address this issue. I have composed a letter you can read or hand to your family, friends, husband, children, or significant other. You can download it from my website at www.femalebraingoneinsane.com. If you wish, you can write your own version. In any event, do it soon. The people you love will appreciate it, and you will feel better because of it.

Dear Loved One,

I am writing to you with a message of apology and explanation for behavior I sincerely regret. The good news is that this is also a message of hope. Hope that I can get better, hope that I can change, and hope for you to have a more stable and balanced person in your life—soon.

I think you know that I have never been comfortable with my mood swings, erratic behavior, my sadness, and occasional outbursts of crying, anger, and remorse. I know that when I am suffering, it causes suffering for all those around me. I have, up to this point, felt powerless over these feelings that simply dominate my actions when I least expect or want them to.

Recently, I decided to do my best to search for answers and help. I found a new book, Female Brain Gone Insane, by a medical professional who has extensive experience treating women who have these very issues. She has helped thousands of women like me. I have read the book carefully and decided to follow the advice and instructions for getting well.

Now, I understand that my brain chemistry is in serious need of renewal and repair. By following the program in the book, I believe

I can bring my brain chemistry back to where it should be, which will eliminate my negative behavior. To get well, I must rebalance my hormonal system, which is compromised and depleted by stress. It will take some time and experimentation, but I expect that we will both see a steady improvement from this point on.

I am now on the right track to recovery and hope you will join and support me as I follow the steps to health and wellness. I would like to discuss the book and share my Emotional Rescue Plan with you. I really need your help with all of this. I need you to believe, as I do, that this book will lead me back to the happy and functional woman you love. I hope you can embrace this new and exciting plan with me. Let's celebrate the hope of a new me with a big hug. I would love that.

With love,

While the topic of dealing with stress is a large one, I hope my suggestions in this chapter have provided you with helpful and useful information. Remember, you are in control and, with the right approach and attitude, it is possible to manage your stress and use it as an opportunity to change, grow, and enhance your entire outlook toward life. Your improved attitude and mood will have a positive effect on your family and circle of friends. Not only will you experience less stress, you will feel healthier, happier, and more energetic, ready to face whatever obstacles come your way.

Part Three

Supplemental Steps for Adrenal and Thyroid Support

Step Five:
Adrenal Health

NOW THAT YOU HAVE IDENTIFIED YOUR emotional type, addressed your brain chemistry, introduced the best mood foods and supplements and effective stress reduction techniques into the program, you'll should feel even more at ease and comfortable in your own skin. If you still feel extremely stressed or suffer from exhaustion, you may want to take a look at your adrenal glands, because long-term stress manifests itself through chemical imbalances of your adrenal hormones. If your adrenal glands are burned out it will take you longer to heal and you may need extra nutritional support. Adrenal fatigue is also an important contributing factor to many health conditions including autoimmune diseases, allergies, and inability to lose weight.

In this chapter, you will learn how your adrenal glands affect your overall health, and if you need adrenal support. This optional step requires that you take a series of tests to determine your adrenal health. With Your Emotional Rescue Plan and pen in hand, fill in the treatment recommendations for Step Five.

By listening to your body, identifying your symptoms, and taking the correct blood and saliva tests you will determine whether your adrenal hormones are too high or too low and what to do about them. You can do some tests at home; others require a visit to the doctor. Remember, adrenal function is just one part of the complex picture that addresses your biochemistry state. Your biochemistry is a constellation of female hormones, brain chemistry, adrenal hormones, and thyroid hormones that dance together. Everything needs to work in inunison to make you feel healthy, strong, and at ease.

Meet Michelle

Michelle was thirty-eight years old when she came to see me. She was climbing the corporate ladder at a local software company and worked about fifty hours a week. She had no children and had lived with an angry, verbally abusive boyfriend for the past six years.

Unhappy with her body, Michelle worked extra hours to pay for liposuction on her belly. She was constantly on the go, getting up at 4:30 AM to hit the gym. She usually skipped breakfast and ate take-out lunch in her car. In the evening, she enjoyed a glass or two of wine with dinner to unwind.

When she came to see me for her first visit she said, "Three months ago, I started having difficulties falling asleep at night. It was as if my brain could not shut down. I felt like something was vibrating inside me, and I could hear my heart pounding hard inside my head. One night I woke up in a horrible panic. My body was shaking out of control and I experienced an overwhelming feeling of doom and fear. I thought I was going to die. My boyfriend took me to the emergency room and the doctor told me I was experiencing a panic attack so he referred me to a psychiatrist, who started me on Prozac. In four weeks, the panic attacks began to diminish, but I still felt terribly anxious and scared, not at all like the Michelle I used to be.

"My boyfriend told me that if I exercised more and lost some weight I would feel better, so I began doing heavy cardio-exercise, running on the treadmill for half an hour daily. I figured it would increase my endorphins and help me feel better. I continued this routine for three months but seemed to get weaker and weaker. Then I got a cold that I still can't seem to shake. I am so exhausted! All I can do is sleep. I feel hopeless and out of control. I also have difficulty waking up in the morning, and my brain feels like a cotton ball. I can't focus, and my memory is shot. I literally hurt from head to toe and even suffer from a sore throat and allergies most every day. I am terrified that my body is slowly shutting down, and soon it will be over. What is going on with me? What do I need to swallow or do to get back to normal again? I'm afraid."

After hearing her story, I knew Michelle was suffering from adrenal burnout. Her body fell into a seemingly never-ending syndrome of fight or flight. Months of intense stress from long hours at the job, lack of sleep, poor nutrition, and an abusive relationship pushed her adrenal glands over the line, and she experienced a cascade of very unpleasant and frightening symptoms. Her body responded as if she was literally running from a tiger on a daily basis. That would wipe out anyone! Remember, the body is only designed to operate optimally during short-lived stress. Once you find a safe cave to regroup and replenish it's over. However, when stress goes on and on, the body can no longer handle it, and women like Michelle suffer with a variety of symptoms.

The chronic stress Michelle initially experienced depleted her serotonin levels and increased her adrenal stress hormones adrenaline and cortisol. After months of continued stress, her serotonin level dropped below the threshold for comfort, and her adrenals were depleted and could no longer produce the adrenal hormones needed for energy and immune defense.

Together, we took a look at her lifestyle and stressors to see what had brought her to this state and what could be changed. Michelle signed up for restorative yoga classes, decided to practice daily meditation, and chose to stop all cardiovascular exercise for three months. It was time to take it easy. I asked her to nap and sleep as long as possible, and to see the nutritionist in my office to improve her eating habits. Michelle started my Basic Supplement Plan (see page 121). She also added the nutritional supplement program for low cortisol (see page 180) so I added 5-HTP in addition to the Basic Supplement Plan to raise her serotonin. Thankfully, Michelle was committed to changing her ways to feel better and find strength and confidence again.

Three months later we had our next visit. She had broken up with her boyfriend and taken in a roommate. She also limited her workweek to a more reasonable forty hours, took yoga two times a week, and began to cook healthier meals. She continued with the psychiatrist who prescribed the Prozac, but because of her improvement, he began to wean her off the drug slowly. Michelle looked alive again and told me her energy had started to come back, and her brain was clear and focused again.

When Stress Is "Good"

Most people believe stress is something to avoid at all costs. However some stress, both physical and emotional, is essential to help your body stay active and alert. "Good" stress is useful; it prepares you for real life dangers and obstacles and gets you through emergencies and tough times. It motivates you to accomplish more and helps you push through what often seems like impossible challenges. However, too much stress for too long often results in emotional and physical problems.

Stress is a highly subjective phenomenon that differs for each person. Ask a group of ten women to explain what stresses them out and they'll give ten different answers. Things like trying to meet a deadline can be stressful for one person while stimulating to another. Many women are seriously addicted to the rush adrenaline (the hormone released by the adrenals under stress) creates in their bodies. They often live packed lives and are constantly on the go. These stress junkies find that their pumped up adrenaline helps them think faster, move faster, and accomplish more. Of course, this kind of lifestyle can only go on so long, because running on adrenaline most of the time eventually leads to burnout and exhaustion.

The Stress Cycle

Hans Selye coined the term *stress* in 1936 as "the non-specific response of the body to any demand for change." Later he redefined it as, "the rate of wear and tear on the body." In a 1951 issue of the *British Medical Journal,* one physician concluded, "Stress, in addition to being itself, was also the cause of itself, and the result of itself." In simple terms: stress breeds stress. It becomes a vicious cycle and can be challenging to resolve. Frequently stress morphs into a way of life rather than just a set of physical symptoms. Remember, symptoms are the key indicators that reveal what is really going on. Your body asks for help by exhibiting symptoms. Your symptoms of stress convey that your body is not receiving the support it needs to sustain the stress and maintain healthy adrenal function.

Fifty Common Signs of Stress

Are you currently experiencing more than three of the following symptoms? If so, you are definitely stressed. Surprised? Of course not. However, you may be surprised to learn how your adrenal glands deal with stress and what you can do to normalize your adrenal hormones.

1. Frequent headaches, jaw clenching, or pain
2. Gritting, grinding teeth
3. Stuttering or stammering
4. Tremors, trembling of lips, hands
5. Neck ache, back pain, muscle spasms
6. Light headedness, faintness, dizziness
7. Ringing, buzzing, or popping sounds
8. Frequent blushing, sweating
9. Cold or sweaty hands, feet
10. Dry mouth, problems swallowing
11. Frequent colds, infections, herpes sores
12. Rashes, itching, hives, "goose bumps"
13. Unexplained or frequent "allergy" attacks
14. Heartburn, stomach pain, nausea
15. Excess belching, flatulence
16. Constipation, diarrhea
17. Difficulty breathing, sighing
18. Sudden attacks of panic
19. Chest pain, palpitations
20. Frequent urination
21. Poor sexual desire or performance

22. Excess anxiety, worry, guilt, nervousness

23. Increased anger, frustration, hostility

24. Depression, frequent or wild mood swings

25. Increased or decreased appetite

26. Insomnia, nightmares, disturbing dreams

27. Difficulty concentrating, racing thoughts

28. Trouble learning new information

29. Forgetfulness, disorganization, confusion

30. Difficulty in making decisions

31. Feeling overloaded or overwhelmed

32. Frequent crying spells or suicidal thoughts

33. Feelings of loneliness or worthlessness

34. Little interest in appearance, punctuality

35. Nervous habits, fidgeting, feet tapping

36. Increased frustration, irritability, edginess

37. Overreaction to petty annoyances

38. Increased number of minor accidents

39. Obsessive or compulsive behavior

40. Reduced work efficiency or productivity

41. Lies or excuses to cover up poor work

42. Rapid or mumbled speech

43. Excessive defensiveness or suspiciousness

44. Problems in communication, sharing

45. Social withdrawal and isolation

46. Constant tiredness, weakness, fatigue

47. Frequent use of over-the-counter drugs

48. Unexplained weight gain or loss

49. Increased smoking, alcohol, or drug use

50. Excessive gambling or impulse buying

Source: The American Institute of Stress

Your Fight or Flight Response

No matter if you experience physical, emotional, or psychological stress, your adrenals become revved up to help out. The adrenals are walnut-sized glands located on top of each kidney. The outer layer of the gland is called the adrenal cortex and produces hormones, including cortisol and dehydroepiandrosterone (DHEA). The center of the gland, known as the medulla, produces epinephrine (which is another word for adrenaline). The master glands in the brain—the hypothalamus and the pituitary—control the adrenals in addition to the thyroid and the ovaries. The stress response triggers the brain to send out large amounts of adrenocorticotropic hormone (ACTH) prompting the adrenals to produce high levels of adrenaline, DHEA, and cortisol.

Cortisol is an important hormone. It helps regulate blood pressure and cardiovascular function, as well as the body's use of proteins, carbohydrates, and fats. Cortisol secretion increases in response to physical and psychological stress during the fight or flight response by giving the body a quick burst of energy to "fight the tiger." Cortisol also increases immunity and lowers the sensitivity to pain. Normally, it is present in the body at higher levels in the morning and at lower levels at night.

DHEA is known as the fountain of youth or mother hormone—as it is a precursor to estrogen, progesterone, testosterone, and cortisone (these hormones are made from DHEA). Our natural DHEA levels typically peak in our twenties and decline with age, which is why there has been considerable interest in DHEA's role in the aging process and whether taking DHEA supplements can slow or reverse some of the signs of aging. In 1994, the *Journal of Clinical Endocrinology and Metabolism* published the first placebo-controlled human study examining the therapeutic effects of DHEA replacement therapy. (*Placebo-controlled* means that some participants received DHEA, while others received fake pills.) The DHEA-takers had more energy, slept better, and handled stress better than the placebo-takers. The researchers concluded, "DHEA will improve the quality of life over a longer period and will postpone some of the unpleasant effects of aging, such as fatigue and muscle weakness." What can the average healthy person expect from DHEA? Many of my patients who took DHEA experienced more energy, could better manage stress, slept better, and were able to lose weight more easily.

Adrenaline (also referred to as epinephrine) increases the fight or flight response of the nervous system. When in the bloodstream, it rapidly prepares the body for action in emergencies. This hormone boosts the supply of oxygen and glucose to the brain and muscles. It increases heart rate and dilates the pupils. It elevates the blood sugar level by increasing the conversion of glycogen to glucose in the liver.

Your Body's Physiological Response to Stress

In a stressful situation, healthy adrenal glands release adrenaline, which makes you more alert and focused. They also release cortisol, which converts protein to energy and releases your stored sugar, known as glycogen, so your body has the fuel needed to respond quickly.

At the same time, your heart rate, respiratory rate, and blood pressure will increase while releasing energy, which tenses your muscles and sharpens your senses. Your digestion slows down and you are primed to fight or flight, whatever is needed. After the threat is gone, your body is designed to return to its normal state. This amazing process was designed to help you survive a serious short-term crisis. The process is not effective for long-term or chronic stress.

Today women are inundated with stress. We are constantly bombarded with technology and stimulation from our cell phones, the Internet, flat screen TVs, iPods, and more. We live in a society where we believe the more we have and do, the happier we will be. Work harder, work longer, do more, earn more, have more, be more. We've become disconnected from nature and friends. Our hands are full with family challenges, chores, impossible schedules, and little down time. We fail to take quality time to unwind or plan and prepare healthy meals, so we end up undernourished and depleted.

All of this stimulation and pressure taxes our adrenals to the max. Although our innate sensitivity to our environment and to the stress we experience makes itself known through symptoms of stress, we try to ignore these signs or self-medicate with alcohol, comfort foods, or tranquilizers. The long-term stress of our daily lives depletes our serotonin storage and causes imbalances in our female hormones, estrogen and progesterone. With these imbalances, even little things will drive us crazy, and suddenly we turn on people who don't deserve it or are really hard on ourselves. We experience Female Brain Gone Insane. As we ignore our body's symptoms, they scream louder and louder, crying for attention and help. Today's uncertain economy and the combination of hopelessness and stress will certainly increase the rate of people suffering from adrenal burnout. Hopefully, we listen before we deplete our energy, emotional well-being, and health.

The same biochemical changes occur in your body for short-term stress as for long-term or chronic stress as well. Your muscles remain tense, your heart and respiration rate are elevated, blood sugar is high, and your digestion slows down. When you finally fall asleep, your mind can continue to spin and you fail to wake up rested, let alone at ease.

With chronic stress, the adrenal glands are constantly on high alert producing high levels of the adrenal hormone cortisol—the hormone that gets the body in gear to fight the tiger. What happens? You experience adrenal burnout, and you feel awful.

Common Stress Triggers

- Caring for aging parents
- Chronic disease
- Food sensitivities
- Death or illness of loved ones
- Demanding boss
- Dieting
- Digestive problems
- Financial pressure
- Hormonal imbalance
- Infections
- Lack of rest
- Lack of sleep
- Malabsorption
- Marital problems
- Noise
- Pain
- Perfectionism
- Skipping meals
- Substance abuse
- Traffic
- Too much input

It's hard to believe, but the majority of my patients experience some form of adrenal imbalance. Either they have cortisol levels that fly through the roof because of short-term stress or suffer from adrenal burnout after long-term stress. According to Dr. James Wilson, author of *Adrenal Fatigue: The 21st Century Stress Syndrome,* an estimated 80 percent of North Americans suffer from adrenal burnout at some point in their lives. Sometimes this condition is temporary and only lasts a few days. However, it can also be debilitating and last for years (or a lifetime if nothing is done about it).

According to a poll commissioned by the New York Academy of Medicine and the National Association of Social Workers, women between the ages of thirty-five and fifty-five are much less likely to be happy than other Americans. This survey of more than 1,000 women (with at least one living parent) found that a mere 20 percent said they were happy compared to 34 percent for the general U.S. population. These women were often caregivers for the elderly and felt the added load of not only managing their own financial challenges, but those of a parent, as well as dealing with lack of time for rest, exercise, and relaxation.

Stress Response Stages

- Stage I—short-term stress response: At the onset of stress, the brain sends out large amounts of adrenocorticotropic hormone (ACTH) prompting the adrenals to produce high levels of adrenaline, DHEA, and cortisol. At the end of this phase DHEA levels start to decrease.
- Stage II—adrenal fatigue: If stress continues, the brain pumps out more ACTH, while the adrenal glands continue to release cortisol and DHEA. Eventually, your adrenal glands cannot adequately meet

the demands put upon them. Cortisol and DHEA start to decline and, as a result, adrenal fatigue sets in. Many women experience symptoms such as fatigue, increased allergies, impaired digestion, fuzzy thinking, depression, salt and carbohydrate cravings, and mood swings.

- Stage III—adrenal burnout: When the adrenals are completely exhausted, tests reveal even lower levels of cortisol, DHEA, and adrenaline. Despite continued stimulation from the brain, the adrenals simply cannot produce adequate hormones. This results in a complete breakdown of the body's ability to cope with stress and can lead to much more serious health concerns including a weakened immune system, fibromyalgia, and chronic fatigue syndrome. The loss of adrenal function can be a long, drawn-out process or a quick and brutal one. A radical event, such a car accident or death of a loved one, can deplete our adrenals quickly. On the other hand, you can experience stressors, such as marital problems and financial pressure, for some time before the adrenals become depleted.

Often, conventional physicians fail to diagnose adrenal fatigue or burnout because in medical school they are taught to look for only extreme adrenal malfunction. They diagnose and treat conditions such as Addison's disease, which occurs when the glands produce far too little cortisol, and Cushing's syndrome, which stems from excessive cortisol production. While Addison's disease is often caused by autoimmune dysfunction, adrenal fatigue is largely caused by stress. It is also less serious than Addison's disease.

Common symptoms in stages I and II of adrenal fatigue include:

- Acne
- Anxiety and irritability

- Blood sugar swings
- Cravings for carbohydrates or sugars
- Depression
- Difficulty falling asleep or interrupted sleep
- Elevated blood pressure
- Elevated blood sugar
- Feeling overwhelmed
- Feeling run down and stressed
- Hair loss
- Impaired memory and cognition
- Intolerance to cold
- Irritable bowel syndrome
- Muscle tension, neck pain
- Nervous breakdown (nervous exhaustion)
- Panic attacks
- Racing thoughts
- Sensitivity to noise
- Weight gain around the middle
- "Wired but tired"

Common symptoms in stage III or adrenal burnout when cortisol and DHEA are quite low and/or depleted:

- Allergies
- Autoimmune problems
- Burnout
- Can't bounce back from stress or illness
- Chemical sensitivity
- Chronic fatigue syndrome (CFS)
- Chronic infections

- Chronic mental and/or physical exhaustion
- Cravings for salt
- Depression
- Fatigue—severe, disabling early morning fatigue
- Feeling best only after 6 PM
- Fibromyalgia
- Lack or loss of strength, generalized weakness
- Need coffee or colas to keep going
- Recurrent, chronic, or slow recovery from respiratory infections
- Rheumatoid arthritis
- Weakness or lack of stamina

Stress and the Sexes

Men and women are hard-wired to react differently to stress, and they require different support to relieve stress. For example, men tend to want to withdraw into their "caves" to relieve stress. They want to forget the problems of their day by watching TV, working on the computer, or puttering around. Women want to interact, connect, and discuss things at length. Why the difference?

In the past, scientists believed women released more cortisol than men, which led to all sorts of nutty theories about why women are so emotional. However, science has proved that there is no consistent difference in cortisol production between men and women.

However, women do produce more of a hormone called oxytocin. This pituitary hormone helps suppress the stress hormone cortisol, which is the hormone that keys the body up for fight or flight. The female hormone estrogen heightens the production of oxytocin, which enhances relaxation, reduces fearfulness, and decreases stress responses.

New studies suggest women release this hormone when they feel acknowledgment, support, and understanding—which, in turn, provide them with a sense of calm and the ability to relax.

As a result, a woman instinctively seeks emotional support in the face of "danger." Psychologist Dr. Shelley Taylor and her UCLA colleagues discovered that females were more likely to deal with stress by "tending and befriending;" that is, nurturing those around them and reaching out to others. We actually increase our oxytocin levels and experience renewed balance and calm when we socialize and talk with our dear ones.

Men also produce oxytocin, but their sex hormone testosterone, produced in high levels when they are under stress, lessens the effects of oxytocin. Instead of "tending and befriending," men are more likely to fight or flee in a stressful situation. Instead of wanting to come home to a sanctuary of love, support, and communication, men head to the "cave" to escape, and in so doing, replenish testosterone levels and get relief.

Take Your Life Back

You will be able to live life again by making the necessary lifestyle and dietary changes to get your adrenals back in shape. It might take some time to get back to normal. Adrenal burnout is not something you can fix overnight. What is most important is to address what got you here in the first place. You've already learned how to balance your female hormones, reduce stress, and change your eating habits through Steps One, Two, Three, and Four. When unavoidable stressors occur, it is best to accept what you cannot change or control and do what you can to be kind to yourself. Read on to learn what you can do to help combat the ravages of stress.

Food Choices Matter

When you experience stress the metabolism of your cells speeds up, rapidly burning up nutrients you absorb from food and supplements. After months of stress, your body uses up its supply of stored nutrients and you become deficient in what you need to function, let alone what you need to heal from your compromised state. It is important to eat nutrition-dense foods, although I know it is difficult to make good eating choices when you're going through periods of stress. Not only is your mind preoccupied with the challenges at hand, but also you often grab the nearest snack to provide some quick energy. That is when it is easy to munch on cookies and chips, or make a quick meal using white bread or pasta.

It is common for women suffering from adrenal fatigue to have gluten sensitivities. Foods such as cereal, oatmeal, bread, and pizza contain gluten. So if you suffer from adrenal fatigue avoid eating gluten completely since any food sensitivities can tax your adrenals and create more problems.

When you experience adrenal burnout, your blood sugar levels can also fluctuate and blood sugar drops can tax the adrenals. To lessen the adrenal burden, never let yourself get too hungry. Eat light meals throughout the day or have a small snack such as almonds, cheese, or an apple every two hours to help keep the blood sugar balanced. Alternatively, consider eating three nutritious meals and two to three small snacks at regular intervals throughout the day.

Mia's Mantra
You are strong

A combination of unrefined carbohydrates (whole grains, beans, and vegetables) with protein (fish, meat, fowl, eggs, and dairy) and good oils (olive, flax oils) is essential to adrenal recovery. Avoid any hydrogenated fats, caffeine, chocolate, white carbohydrates, such as white bread, and junk foods. If you have cravings for salt, get your salt-shaker out and use it in moderation. Unless you have been diagnosed with high blood pressure (the majority of people with adrenal fatigue have low blood pressure, not high) it may be beneficial to add moderate amounts of salt to your diet. To learn more about what to eat to support your stamina, mood, and health, review Step Four starting on page 137.

A Warning About Exercise

Many studies confirm the benefits of exercise, however, it may be time for you to take a break from it. Your nervous system is already in high gear from stress and doing too much. Ask yourself:

- Do I feel worse after exercise?
- Does exercise make me feel exhausted?
- Am I gaining weight no matter how much I exercise?

If you answered yes to any of these questions, exercise is just not good for you right now. If you are in the first stage of adrenal burnout with high levels of the stress hormone cortisol, exercise will actually increase your level of cortisol. High cortisol causes weight gain especially around the middle. So, in this situation, exercise may add to your stress, increasing the risk for stroke and heart attacks, and causing you to gain weight. In the third phase of adrenal burnout, you become exhausted. At this point, your body needs rest. Exercise will just tax those tired adrenal glands even more, and you will end up in complete exhaustion.

Test Your Adrenal Levels

Because symptoms are not the best indicator of adrenal function, I strongly encourage you to have your levels of cortisol and DHEA-S tested. DHEA-S (DHEA sulfate) is the best test for evaluating your DHEA level. It is important to test not only your overall levels of cortisol, but also to have a test that tracks the way it cycles throughout the day.

I believe a saliva test provides the most accurate results to determine adrenal health. Your doctor can provide you with a kit of tubes for colleting your saliva, or you can order the kits on your own. To test the way your cortisol levels cycle throughout the day you should take saliva samples four times during the same day—at 8 AM, noon, 4 PM, and 10 PM. Normally, levels are high in the morning and taper off by the afternoon. Saliva testing is inexpensive and easy to do at home. The following labs provide saliva test kits for a minimum cost of $80–$150. Each lab will provide you with their reference levels (what is considered normal levels) of cortisol and DHEA and a sample report for you to view.

You can order the Stress Check test on your own from Body Balance at www.body balance.com. If you like, have your doctor order an Adrenal Stress Panel test for you from LABRIX at www.labrix.com or the Adrenocortex Stress Profile test from Genova Diagnostics at www.genova diagnostics.com. ZRT Laboratory at www. zrtlab.com can provide DHEA-S and cortisol testing through your doctor.

Get ready to refer back to Step Five of Your Emotional Rescue Plan worksheet to fill in your results and recommendations for adrenal support.

After receiving your test results, you will know the status of your adrenals. If your cortisol tested higher than normal, it means your adrenals are making a lot of cortisol to keep up with the demands of your stressful life. Your body still thinks it is constantly being chased by a tiger. DHEA-S levels usually parallel cortisol levels and tend to be high in the initial phases of stress.

If your cortisol tested lower than normal, it means your adrenals are being exhausted and can no longer keep up with the demands of your stressful life. When cortisol levels start dropping below normal, often the DHEA-S levels will test low as well. This is when the body starts screaming to you, "stop, lay down, rest, breath," and you start experiencing common symptoms of adrenal burnout.

Your Emotional Rescue Plan for Adrenal Health

Whether your test results reveal your cortisol levels are too high or too low, it means you are currently under too much stress or have been for a long time. Taking a look at your lifestyle should be your first priority when it comes to adrenal support. You have just read Step Four: Stress-buster and Life-improvement Techniques, and I encourage you practice some of the stress relievers presented there. My chief recommendations include:

- Remove stressors. It is important you face what got you into the trenches of imbalance in the first place.
- Change the way your body responds to stress.
- Balance your biochemistry, make sure your female hormones are balanced.

Nutritional Supplements for Adrenal Health

If test results show your cortisol levels are too high take:

Type of supplement	Dose	When
Seriphos (phosphorlated serine) by Inter Plexus, Inc.	1 capsule	1 to 4 times daily

Seriphos contains serine phosphate as a calcium and magnesium derivative in a base of calcium and magnesium ethanolamine phosphate. This supplement works by reducing ACTH, the pituitary hormone that orders your adrenals to release cortisol under stress, therefore you will end up with less circulating cortisol.

Seriphos is best taken one hour before the time of day when your cortisol levels are elevated above normal. Your saliva test results will give you four different levels throughout the day. Seriphos should only be taken for one to two months. You don't want to turn your adrenals down too low. Once you have used Seriphos for one to two months have your cotisol levels rechecked. Don't take Seriphos if you are pregnant or breast-feeding.

Type of supplement	Dose	When
Theanine Serine with Relora by Source Naturals	2 capsules	1 to 3 times daily

This product contains the amino acid L-theanine, to support relaxing brain wave activity, and taurine to ease tension, as well as the calming neurotransmitter GABA. It also features magnesium to support muscle and nerve relaxation, and calming holy basil leaf extract and Relora to soothe away the tension in your body gently. Do not take this product if you already are taking these amino acids for your Emotional Type.

If your test results show your cortisol levels are too low take:

Type of supplement	Dose
Vitamin C	2000–4000 mg sustained release
Vitamin E with mixed tocopherols	800 IU
Niacin as inositol hexaniacinate	125–150 mg
B₆	150 mg
B₅ (pantothenic acid)	1200–1500 mg
Magnesium citrate	400–1200 mg

Please note: This is the total daily amount of these nutrients including what is in Mia's Basic Supplement Plan.

Other supplements recommended for low cortisol levels. The dosages vary among manufacturers:

- Licorice root extract
- Ashwaganda Root
- Rhodiola Rosea
- Desiccated Whole Adrenal Glandular

For suggested brands and products, visit www.femalebraingoneinsane.com

If your DHEA-S tested lower than normal, take the following supplement in addition to Mia's Basic Supplement Plan:

Type of supplement	Dose	When
7-Keto DHEA	25 mg	Once daily with meals

7-Keto stands for 3-acetyl-7-oxo-dehydroepiandrosterone, which is a naturally occurring metabolite of DHEA, a hormone produced by the adrenal gland. DHEA is the most abundant of the adrenal hormones and functions as a precursor for many important sex hormones, such as estrogen and testosterone.

The most fundamental difference between DHEA and 7-Keto DHEA is that 7-Keto DHEA is already converted DHEA, so, it will not spike estrogen and testosterone, as does DHEA alone. 7-Keto is a clinically studied, safe form of DHEA. It is associated with a variety of essential human functions like weight loss, immunology, memory, and aging.

Your Time Frame for Adrenal Recovery

Please take your treatment plan seriously and be patient. Your adrenals will recover and you will start feeling healthier and like yourself again. Give yourself some time to rebuild and restore your adrenal function. Continue to practice your lifestyle changes and take your supplements with these periods in mind:

- 6 to 9 months for minor adrenal fatigue
- 12 to 18 months for moderate fatigue
- Up to 24 months for severe adrenal fatigue

I recommend you repeat your adrenal saliva test after following the protocol for about two to there months. Once your levels are normal, you can stop the recommend supplements.

Step Six: The Thyroid Connection

THIS CHAPTER EDUCATES YOU ABOUT your thyroid: how it works, and how it responds to stress. You will also learn about the tests to take to determine your thyroid function. Then you'll find out how to modify your diet and lifestyle, as well as what supplements and medication might be necessary so you feel and function at your best. You might want to read this chapter if you have a family history of a sluggish thyroid or if you still suffer symptoms of brain fog and fatigue or feel cold much of the time.

By the way, I address only under-active thyroid in this chapter and will not talk about hyperthyroidism, or over-active thyroid. Why? Hyperthyroidism has typically severe symptoms such as rapid heartbeat, nervousness, and weight loss, and your doctor can easily diagnose and effectively treat it. If you have the symptoms mentioned above, please see your doctor right away.

Mia's
Mantra
You have the
power to
change

Meet Kristine

As a thirty-six-year-old accountant, Kristine had no children and lived with her fiancée. She suffered from a long history of severe migraines, as well as constipation, fatigue, and mild depression. When she came to see me she told me she rarely felt up to par. When I touched her hands and feet they felt cold as ice cubes! Even in the summer months, Kristine said she had to sleep in thick socks to keep warm. Although her work required detail-oriented thinking, Kristen confessed she couldn't think very clearly and she found it more and more difficult to crunch numbers.

I ran a thyroid blood test, which showed Kristen was suffering from an underactive thyroid. Kristen started taking thyroid hormones and she also visited a nutritionist to learn what food supported healthy thyroid function. When she returned six weeks later, she reported her headaches were entirely gone and her energy and focus were better than ever. "This feels like a miracle! The pill I swallow is so tiny but it has made such a huge improvement in my overall life!" Her depression had also lifted and her intolerance to cold had improved. Five weeks later, I did a repeat test of her thyroid panel and all of her levels had returned to normal.

Just like Kristine, you could be one of more than 59 million Americans suffering from the frequently misdiagnosed condition called hypothyroidism. This condition is very common in the perimenopausal and postmenopausal years. Hypothyroidism means you have an underactive or sluggish thyroid gland, which can really make you feel lousy.

Your thyroid is a tiny but powerful butterfly-shaped gland in your neck. It weighs less than one ounce and affects every single cell and hormone in your body. Its main purpose is to run your body's metabolism, and it regulates how many calories you burn and how warm you feel. When your body lacks sufficient thyroid hormone, everything in your body and mind slows down. Like Kristen, you may feel cold or constipated; and your brain might feel sluggish so you can't think too clearly. An underactive thyroid can lead to weight gain, depression, heavy menstrual cycles, and a low libido. Recent studies indicate that depressed patients who were unresponsive to antidepressant medications felt significantly better after taking thyroid hormones in addition to an antidepressant.

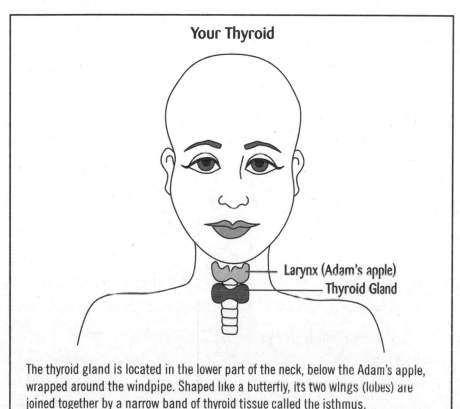

Your Thyroid

Larynx (Adam's apple)
Thyroid Gland

The thyroid gland is located in the lower part of the neck, below the Adam's apple, wrapped around the windpipe. Shaped like a butterfly, its two wings (lobes) are joined together by a narrow band of thyroid tissue called the isthmus.

Your Thyroid: A Valuable Hormone Dance Partner

Remember, healthy thyroid function is just one part of the biochemical synergy that leads to neuroendocrine well-being. Your overall health relies on the interrelationship of your female hormones, brain chemistry, adrenal hormones, and thyroid hormones. When all four systems dance together and maintain their ideal balance, you feel good. However, when a disruption occurs in the equilibrium, you can experience physical and emotional distress.

Now that you have addressed your adrenals, it's time to focus on your thyroid gland. It is important to treat your adrenal condition first—before tackling a thyroid problem. So make sure to work through Step Five before starting this step.

Here are some other examples of how brain chemistry and other hormonal systems affect your thyroid and vice versa.

• Low serotonin causes low thyroid.
• Low thyroid causes low serotonin.
• High cortisol and high adrenaline causes low thyroid.
• Too high estrogen blocks thyroid.

Symptoms of Low Thyroid

A variety of symptoms are associated with hypothyroidism. If you suffer from three or more of the following conditions, your thyroid may be involved.

• Allergies that suddenly appear or get worse
• Anxiety
• Body aches

- Brittle nails
- Cold hands and feet
- Constipation
- Depression
- Difficulty losing weight
- Dry hair or hair loss
- Elevated levels of LDL (the "bad" cholesterol)
- Fatigue
- Fertility problems
- Fluid retention
- Headaches
- Heavy menstrual flow
- Hoarseness
- Irregular menstrual cycles
- Loss of outer third of the eyebrow
- Low libido
- Memory loss, fuzzy thinking, difficulty following conversation or train of thought
- Muscle or joint aches
- Pale skin
- Palpitations
- Persistent cold sores, boils, or breakouts
- PMS
- Poor concentration
- Poor memory
- Lack of motivation
- Puffiness in face and extremities
- Tingling sensation in wrists and hands that mimics carpal tunnel syndrome
- Weakness

How Does Your Thyroid Work?

The hypothalamus in the brain sends a message to the pituitary gland by releasing thyroid-releasing hormone (TRH). In turn, the pituitary gland releases thyroid-stimulating hormone (TSH) to stimulate the thyroid gland to release the thyroid hormones. The thyroid makes and releases two main hormones into the bloodstream called thyroxine (T4) and triiodothyronine (T3). The T4 converts to T3, which is the biologically active form of the two thyroid hormones.

The thyroid works like the thermostat in your house. If it makes just the right amount of hormones, it keeps the temperature just right. If the thyroid is too active and produces too much T4 and T3, it is like having a thermostat that's set too high, so the house gets overheated. If the thyroid is not active enough, the thermostat will be set too low and the house will be too cold—which is what happens with hypothyroidism.

The more you allow stress to run your life, the more inefficient your thyroid becomes and the fewer hormones it will make. The stress hormone cortisol blocks the conversion of T4 to T3 leading to less T3 in your system. If your T3 hormone is not produced in proper amounts, the rest of your body will not function well. It is the lack of T3 that makes you hypothyroid.

The Thyroid Testing Controversy

In the past, your doctor may have tested your thyroid and told you, "Your thyroid tests are fine. Nothing is wrong." You may have walked out of the office confused. You may have wondered, *Why do I feel this way? I know something isn't right.* Many of the thyroid tests performed in doctors' offices today are poor measures of thyroid function. There are several reasons for this problem. First, the majority of health care practitioners, including endocrinologists, rely solely on one test known as TSH (Thyroid Stimulating Hormone) as the primary test or gold standard for diagnosing and managing most thyroid conditions. They often exclude other important testing that measures Free T4, Free T3 ("free" means bioavailable or active) and thyroid antibodies levels. In addition, test results are interpreted using a reference or normal range that is too rigid, which places people with abnormally high levels of TSH in the normal range. Remember, high TSH means low thyroid (hypothyroidism). By erroneously categorizing relatively high TSH hormone levels as normal, the medical community leaves millions of people undiagnosed who continue to suffer symptoms from low thyroid.

The recent Colorado Thyroid Disease Prevalence Study found that 13 million Americans may be unaware of or undiagnosed for their underactive thyroid condition because they fall within what is considered the normal range of the TSH test result category. Fortunately, the American Association of Clinical Endocrinologists has revised this guideline, but many labs and health care practitioners continue to use the old standard.

In addition, most traditional doctors do not test for the active thyroid hormone T3 because they believe the body converts all the T4 it needs into T3. It is my belief that this misnomer results in even more undiagnosed and untreated cases of hypothyroidism. This is why I strongly encourage women to undergo a complete series of thyroid tests to make sure they are well informed and treated properly.

Recommended Thyroid Tests

Although I believe a blood test is the most accurate measure of thyroid function, your basal body temperature can serve as a general measure, and checking it is easy to do at home. Because the thyroid controls your basal body temperature, your temperature can gauge how much T3 is active within the cells. A low basal temperature suggests a slow metabolism or low thyroid function.

To see if your temperature suggests that you may have low thyroid function, follow these steps for an accurate reading:

- In the morning before you get out of bed, place the thermometer under your tongue.
- Remain as still as possible resting with your eyes closed.
- Record the temperature for at least three consecutive mornings, preferably at the same time of the day. To get an accurate reading, menstruating women need to check their temperature on the second, third, and fourth day of menstruation.
- If your average temperature is below 97.8° Fahrenheit, then there is a good chance you have a low functioning thyroid.

Blood Tests for Your Thyroid

If your temperature suggests you have low thyroid function, I recommend you follow up with a blood test to get an accurate picture of your thyroid function. You'll need to check the levels of the pituitary TSH hormone, in addition to the actual thyroid hormones T3 (free and reverse) and T4. I also recommend thyroid peroxidase (TPO) and thyroid antibody (anti-thyroid AB) tests to determine if an autoimmune disease is causing your low thyroid function. This may sound like a lot of testing, however, you will benefit from knowing as much as you can about the health of this powerful gland.

Recommended Tests:

1. Thyroid Stimulating Hormone—TSH

2. FT4 (free T4)

3. FT3 (free T3)

4. Reverse T3

5. Thyroid Peroxidase Antibodies (TPO)

6. Anti-thyroid Antibodies

Ask your doctor to order the above tests for you or order them yourself through the websites that follow. Each lab will provide you with normal values.

My Med Lab www.mymedlab.com

1. Purchase testing online, or by phone, and then visit one of nearly 2,000 local Patient Service Centers (PSC) in your neighborhood.

2. Once samples are drawn, results are securely uploaded to your private personal health record (PHR), most within 24 to 48 hours.

3. A notification email is sent when results have been released and are ready for review.

4. Then simply log into their PHR account at MyMedLab (with your user name and password you created) to view your results. Each result includes a brief explanation and a direct link to the National Library of Medicine for more detailed result information.

Life Extension Foundation www.lef.org/bloodtest/

1. Call 1-800-208-3444 or order online, and they will send you a requisition form.

2. Visit one of the LabCorp draw stations closest to you to have your blood drawn. You will receive a list of the three labs closest to you via mail.

3. Blood test results may take up to two weeks to be completed. Results will be mailed upon completion of all tests.

4. Members are able to request their own blood tests and have the opportunity to discuss the results of these tests with one of Life Extension's doctors.

Thyroid Laboratory Values and Interpretation

Test name	Normal Range	Interpretation
TSH	0.3 to 3.0 IU/mL (as of 2003)	Less than 0.3 can indicate possible hyperthyroidism. Levels higher than 3.0 are considered indicative of hypothyroidism. Note: These are guidelines were revised and adopted in 2003 by the American Association of Clinical Endocrinologists. Be aware that many labs and practitioners do not interpret results using these revised guidelines.
Free T4 (free thyroxine)	0.7 to 2.0 ng/dL	Less than 2.3 is considered indicative of possible hypothyroidism. Over 4.2 can indicate hyperthyroidism.
Free T3 (free triiodothyronine)	2.3 to 4.2 pg/mL	Less than 2.3 can indicate hypothyroidism. Levels higher than 4.2 can indicate hyperthyroidism.
TPO-Ab (thyroid peroxidase antibodies)	less than 2 IU/mL	Elevated levels can indicate autoimmune disease of the thyroid.
TGA (thyroglobulin antibodies)	less than 1 IU/mL	Elevated levels can indicate autoimmune disease of the thyroid.

Note: Reference values can vary from lab to lab. Always check to find out what the specific normal ranges are at your lab. The ranges should be listed on the lab report.

Treat Your Thyroid with Love

Besides taking supplements or medication for your thyroid, follow my practical advice:

- Eliminate stressors whenever possible.
- Make sure to continue with Mia's Basic Supplement Plan as the recommended supplements contain several nutrients essential for proper thyroid function.
- Enjoy apricots, dates, egg yolk, parsley, potatoes, prunes, raw seeds, whole grains, and seafood to support thyroid function.
- Avoid foods such as saturated fats, sugars, white flour, Brussels sprouts, cabbage, broccoli, kale, mustard greens, peaches, and pears. These foods contain certain chemicals that can suppress the thyroid function and the normal production of thyroid hormones.
- Avoid the common causes of thyroid problems, such as heavy metals and environmental toxins. Try to eat organic foods; don't eat fish more than two to three times per week; avoid amalgam fillings; take nutritional supplements that have been verified for quality and purity to insure that they are free from pesticides, bacteria, and heavy metals; filter your water; and avoid insecticides as much as possible.
- If you are sensitive to any foods avoid them because they can interfere with your thyroid function.

If you are suffering from either low or high levels of cortisol, you may not be able to tolerate any type of thyroid medication, in particular T4 and T3 combinations. It is advisable to have your adrenal function evaluated before starting thyroid replacement therapy.

Thyroid Hormone Supplements

Type	Brand Names
Desiccated animal thyroid commonly called natural thyroid.	Armour Thyroid, Nature-Throid, Westhroid

Synthetic supplements, yet bioidentical to the hormones made by the human thyroid:

Type	Brand Names
T4 Only	Synthroid, Levoxyl, Levothyroxine
T3 only	Cytomel
T4 T3 combination	Thyrolar

Doctors most often prescribe a synthetic T4-only replacement such as Synthroid and Levoxyl because of the erroneous assumption that the body will convert the T4 to the biologically active form of T3. Many patients who take the T4-only preparations will continue to suffer from low thyroid because their T3 levels remain low despite T4 replacement therapy.

Desiccated thyroid or thyroid extract is a thyroid hormone derived from pig's thyroids, which has been used as a treatment for hypothyroidism since the late 1800s. This product is sometimes referred to as "natural thyroid" or "natural thyroid hormones," because it is not the synthetic variety. Some doctors claim desiccated thyroid preparations have consistency problems or are dangerous, despite the fact that these preparations have been the treatment of choice for many years. How do you know which type of thyroid hormone replacement is safest and best for you?

In *Thyroid Power,* holistic practitioner Dr. Richard Shames, who has treated thyroid conditions for a quarter century, offers the following advice that I support:

> In 25 years of practice, I have found that it doesn't necessarily matter which kind of thyroid hormone you start with so much, as which kind you end up with after trying several different types to see which one works best for you. Initially, I typically recommend whatever type they have either heard about, have a "gut-feeling" about, know family members who have a good response to a particular kind of medicine, or have a philosophical inclination for one kind or another. Sometimes it is the combination of two or three of the above medicines that proves to be the magic solution for a particular person. If the initial item tried does not give 85–95 percent improvement, I then encourage the person to either add something to their first choice product or discontinue it and start something new. It is my firm belief that the state of the art in finding the optimal medicine is still trial and error.

Mia's Tips for Taking your Thyroid Medication

1. Take your thyroid hormone on an empty stomach, at least half an hour before eating to allow for maximum absorption.
2. Don't change your fiber-eating habits. If you do, get your thyroid rechecked because it may change your results.
3. If you take iron or calcium supplements or antacids, consume them at least two or three hours apart from your thyroid medication. They can interfere with thyroid hormone absorption
4. Check on interactions with other medications. Cholesterol

lowering drugs, antibiotics, Topamax, beta-blockers and, anti-depressants are just a few that can make thyroid medications more or less effective. Go online to Drug Interaction Checker, at http://www.drugs.com/drug_interactions.html for more information.

Thyroid Factoids:

- Treat possible adrenal conditions before starting thyroid replacement.
- The thyroid affects every cell and hormone in your body.
- Stress blocks thyroid function.
- The most active thyroid hormone is T3.
- THS by itself is not a reliable test of thyroid function.

Make sure to fill in Step Six of Your Emotional Rescue Plan now that you know what to do to ensure your thyroid is healthy and functioning at an optimal level. Ask your doctor to perform the tests that I recommend if you have not had them done on your own.

Afterword: How to Keep Your Emotional Rescue Plan Current

By NOW YOU HAVE FOLLOWED Your Emotional Rescue Plan for several weeks, and I know you are feeling more grounded and in control of your emotions. I've provided you with a lot of information to assimilate and many supplements to take. If you are a tad overwhelmed, don't worry! By reading this book and following Your Emotional Rescue Plan you've demonstrated your courage and tenacity to change your biochemistry and your life. I want to congratulate you on your efforts and your success. At last, your brain chemistry and hormones are finally dancing in unison, or well on their way. I hope that your world is now glowing in living color and it looks and feels three-dimensional again. Now you can relate to yourself and others in a happier way. Open your heart and tap into your true goodness, the beauty of life, and ability to live it to the fullest.

As women, we are caretakers. We care about everyone and everything. We nurture those around us. In addition, we feel the pain of others and lately, the discomforts of our own bodies and minds. *Female Brain Gone Insane* primarily focuses on our discomfort more than our pleasure. Obviously, it is a guidebook for feeling healthy again. However, the whole spirit behind this book is to help you get to a place where you can finally relax, feel contentment, self-acceptance, and joy. The root of happiness, as I see it, is in a balanced biochemistry combined with the wisdom that comes from that balanced place. Only when your brain chemistry is balanced will you be able to do the emotional and spiritual work that it takes to grow into the rest of your life with grace.

Mia's Mantra

You are a wonderful human being

Life is about making changes. Therefore, as you move through life and heal, I encourage you to trust yourself to adjust your plan according to how you feel. As you enter into a new hormonal phase or face new life stressors, your need for hormonal and brain chemistry support (as well as diet shifts and lifestyle activities) will change. That means you are now in charge of updating Your Emotional Rescue Plan.

Change Your Plan with Your Mood

As time goes by, you will need to adjust Your Emotional Rescue Plan depending on how you feel. Remember, it is a change in your biochemistry that will change the way you feel. Bumps in the road—such as kids going off to college, aging parents, challenging teenagers, moves, and death of loved ones—all create stress that will change your biochemistry.

If you stop feeling at the top of your game, use your Monthly Symptom Tracker to record how you feel, then:

1. Go back to Troubleshooting for All of the Emotional Types in Step Two (page 111). There you will find out how to adjust your supplements based on how you feel.
2. Revisit Step Four for suggestions on how to reduce the stress in your life.

Change Your Plan as
Your Hormone Phase Changes

As you age, your hormonal status will naturally change and you will transition into a new hormonal phase. The following changes might indicate that you have transitioned in to a new hormonal phase.

- Your periods are getting heavier or lighter.
- Your periods have become irregular.
- You are taking progesterone without estrogen and you are starting to feel odd or depressed on the progesterone.
- You are taking progesterone without estrogen and you are starting to experience typical menopausal symptoms such as hot flashes, night sweats, insomnia, and crying spells (see more symptoms of menopause on page 86–87).

Initially, in the PMS and perimenopausal phases, you will just need progesterone to help you feel better (in addition to taking the supplements for your brain chemistry, improving your diet, and lowering your stress), but as you enter into menopause you will need estrogen and probably some testosterone as well. Review Step One periodically, and follow the protocols given for your new hormonal phase.

Change Your Plan as
Your Adrenal Hormones Improve

Adrenal recovery does not happen overnight. If your adrenal hormone cortisol tested very low it can take up to a year, sometimes two, to recover completely. Your adrenals will recover, and you will start feeling healthier and like yourself again. Give yourself some time to rebuild and restore your adrenal function. Continue to practice your lifestyle changes and take your supplements with these time frames in mind:

- 6 to 9 months for minor adrenal fatigue
- 12 to 18 months for moderate fatigue
- Up to 24 months for severe adrenal fatigue

I recommend you repeat your adrenal saliva test every two to three months. Once your levels are normal, you can stop the recommend supplements.

Take an Honest Look Inside

Now that you have found a balanced biochemistry and feel good, stable, and more in control, ask these critical questions: *How did I initially end up in such a difficult emotional place? Why did I feel so bad? What really has to change in my life to find long-term emotional well-being and contentment?* Take an honest look at yourself. Consider how you have been thinking, feeling, and acting. Remember, stress contributes to the degree of distress and intensifies symptoms. It contributes a huge piece to the puzzle of imbalance that pushes you over the edge and into the trenches. Perhaps you are a perfectionist. Maybe you are a people-pleaser and bend over backwards to get approval from others. On the other hand, perhaps you are an overachiever and just have too much on your plate. Possibly you surround yourself with people who drain your energy.

Often, when you are unhappy, you may think, *If only one or two things in my life would change, everything would be fine. If only I lost ten pounds, got a new car, remodeled the kitchen, I would be happy.* The list can go on and on as you set conditions for happiness. All of us yearn for *more.* This is a form of insanity and a major stress creator! You have to let go of this voice. Give yourself a break. Only when you stop pushing will you be able to find some peace, keep your biochemistry in balance, and devote more of yourself to what you know is truly important. Here is a message from my heart that I believe is very meaningful and will encourage you to live more in the moment:

As they say, one day at a time. It's useless to reproach yourself for whatever happened before this very moment and futurizing sets ups, unncessary worry, and apprehension.

You know this. You've experienced it way too many times. I want to encourage you to live life today. Easy to say, of course, but crucial and wise. Make your day alive, vibrant, loving, and if possible beautiful. And if you can only breathe, forgive yourself, and move moment to moment, do so with as much gratitude as possible.

Mia's Tips for Daily Living

- Spend more time with friends, family, and loved ones. Without them, everything means nothing.
- Pay attention to the small details that you enjoy in your everyday life.
- Walk in nature, spend time in the garden, paint, sing, or just laugh out loud.
- Share what you have with those less fortunate.
- Tell those who mean so much to you how much you care and love them.
- Never take one single breath for granted.
- Start your day showing gratitude. Say to yourself as you wake up in the morning, "I am so grateful for _____" and name at least three things.

Let Go

Recently, a study reported on women who lived one hundred years or more. These fortunate women shared two important lifestyle characteristics: they engaged in some form of physical activity, and they had all learned how to "let go." Not just once, but over and over again.

I have had the privilege of seeing women of all ages grow and thrive during my many years of practice. I have learned so much from those who seem to know how to open new doors, but they also know how to close other doors behind them. We must move forward, and we must accept life's difficulties. As women, we are complex and sensitive beings that have the wisdom, resiliency, and spirit that allows us to move through life with true grace. As we age, we must learn to accept loss and change—to let go—while cherishing each day for the beautiful gift it is.

In each stage of life, there are wonderful experiences one can savor and valuable insights one can absorb. Every new decade brings with it wisdom, transformation, and growth, as well as ends and beginnings. I remember the last time I breastfed my daughter. I cried when I was doing it because I knew it was the last time. She was ready to stop. Never again would I have a child at my breast. I had to close that door. And I did. You can also learn to let go—one day, one experience at a time. Appreciate each new milestone you reach. Take pleasure in the delights of your age, whether you are in your 20s to 40s, 50s to 70s, or 80s to 100s.

Message of Hope

My goal has been to hold your hand and rescue you from the trenches of hopelessness and despair through these pages filled with information, inspiration, and support. I am confident you are no longer falling apart. With this book's help, you have saved yourself and now stand on solid, safe ground. You are ready to reclaim your joyous and happy life.

Although you have reached the end of this book, it is not the end of your journey. In many ways, it is the beginning of a new and more vital chapter of your life—a new you. You can listen to your body and brain and know how to help yourself. You can articulate how you feel and know your true needs. Moreover, you have the tools to maintain your sanity and experience a fulfilling life. I have no doubt you now know what to do to take care of yourself. At last, you are strong, confident, and able.

It is time I let go. My job is done. It has been my pleasure and an honor to help you.

Come to the edge, Life said.
They said: We are afraid.
Come to the edge, Life said.
They came to the edge.
Life pushed them.
And they flew!

—GUILLAUME APOLLINAIRE
1870–1918

Resources for Sanity

THE FOLLOWING IS A LIST OF useful websites, tools, and organizations where you can find more information or seek additional help for your personalized emotional rescue plan.

Health Care Practitioner Referrals

It can be difficult to find a health care practitioner who is willing to work with you as a partner in your health care. The following resources can help you find a practitioner familiar with bioidentical hormone replacement therapy, amino acid therapy for neurotransmitter function, adrenal support, and thyroid hormone replacement.

Female Brain Gone Insane
www.femalebraingoneinsane.com

I have created a very informative and interactive website providing you with the following:

- Blogs.
- Forums.

- Referrals to health care practitioners who have been trained by me.
- Vitamin store.
- Webinars and teleconferences.
- Follow new research on bioidentical hormones and more.
- Down load and print the following forms:
  - Your Monthly Symptom Tracker
  - Your Emotional Rescue Plan
  - Letter to you Health Care Practitioner
  - Letter to Your Loved One
- And much more. . . .

The Center for Hormonal and Nutritional Balance, Inc.
and the office of Mia Lundin, R.N.C., N.P.
Call if you would like a private phone consult or to schedule a visit.
601 E. Arrellaga Street, Suite 201
Santa Barbara, CA 93103
(805) 882-1956
www.hormonesandnutrition.com

The Institute for Functional Medicine
4411 Pt. Fosdick Drive NW, Suite 305
P.O. Box 1697
Gig Harbor, WA 98335
(800) 228-0622
www.functionlamedicine.org

American College for Advancement in Medicine (ACAM)
8001 Irvine Center Drive, Suite 825
Irvine, CA 92618
(800) 532-3688
www.acam.org

American College for Advancement in Medicine
P.O. Box 3427
Laguna Hills, CA 92654
(800) 532-3688
www.acam.org

American Association of Naturopathic Physicians
601 Valley St., Ste. #105
Seattle, WA 98109
(206) 298-0126
www.naturopathic.org/welcome.html

American Holistic Medical Association
Resources for natural HRT.
23366 Commerce Park, Suite 101B
Beachwood, Ohio 44122
(216) 292-6644
www.holisticmedicine.org

American Academy of Anti-Aging Medicine (A4M)
1510 W. Montana Street
Chicago, IL 60614
USA
(773) 528-1000
www.worldhealth.net

International Society for Orthomolecular Medicine
www.orthomolecular.org

Find a thyroid specialist who prescribes Armour Thyroid:
www.thyroid-info.com/topdrs/armour.htm

Find a licensed Biofeedback Practitioner:
Biofeedback Certification Institute of America.
www.bcia.org

Find a licensed NLP Practitioner:
The NLP Database & Practitioners Resource Directory
www.nlp-practitioners.com

The NLP and Coaching Institute of California:
www.nlpca.com

Find a licensed Acupuncturist:
The American Association of Acupuncture Oriental Medicine
(AAAOM)
www.aaaomonline.org/45000.asp

How to Find a Compounding Pharmacy

The easiest way to locate a compounding pharmacy is to contact one of the following associations:

Professional Compounding Centers of America, Inc. (PCCA)
9901 S. Wilcrest
Houston, TX 77099
(800) 331-2498
www.pccarx.com

International Academy of Compounding Pharmacists (IACP)
4638 Riverstone Blvd.
Missouri City, TX 77459
(800) 927-4227
www.iacprx.org

National Association of Compounding Pharmacies (NACP)
4015 River Road
Amarillo, TX 79108
(800) 687-7850

Pharmacy Compounding Accreditation Board
1100 15th Street, NW
Washington, DC 20005
(866) 377-5104
http://www.pcab.org/find-a-pharmacy.shtml#ca

Women's International Pharmacy
Women's International Pharmacy has put together a very compre-
   hensive dosing table representing some of the more frequently
   prescribed regimens for women in menopause and some alternatives. This dosing table can be printed and brought to your doctor.
Here you can also "Find A Doctor Who Prescribes Bioidentical
   Hormones."
http://www.womensinternational.com

Laboratories Where You Can
Order Your Own Tests

Blood tests

My Med Lab
This lab was designed to put you, the consumer, back in control of your
   health, allowing you to make informed health care choices for
   yourself.
https://www.mymedlab.com/tests.php

Life Extension Foundation

Members are able to request their own blood tests and have the opportunity to discuss the results of these tests with one of Life Extension's doctors.

http://www.lef.org/bloodtest/

Saliva Hormone Testing

Body Balance

www.bodybalance.com

ZRT Laboratory

www.zrtlab.com

Laboratories That Require a Requisition from a Doctor

Female, Adrenal, and Thyroid Hormones

Labrix

(877) 656-9596

www.labrix.com

Genova Diagnostics

Genova Diagnostics

63 Zillicoa Street

Asheville, NC 28801

(800) 522-4762

www.genovadiagnostics.com

Metametrix Clinical Laboratory
3425 Corporate Way
Duluth, GA 30096
(800) 221-4640
www.metametrix.com

Neurotransmitter and Adrenal Testing

NeuroScience Inc.
373 280th Street
Osceola, WI 54020
(888) 342-7272
www.neurorelief.com

Sanesco
1010 Merrimon Ave.
Asheville, NC 28804
(866) 670-5705
www.sanesco.net

Where to Buy Brain-mood Food, Supplements, and Nonprescription Bioidentical Hormones

You can either go to your health food store or shop online for the progesterone, food, and supplements you need to get back to sanity. Make sure you pick products produced by companies that assure product quality and purity. You will be able to find professional grade nutritional supplements at:

www.femalebraingoneinsane.com

You can also ask your healthcare provider to order professional grade products through the following companies:

Emerson Ecologics
Bedford, NH
(800) 654-4432
Redlands, CA
(800) 824-2434
www.emersonecologics.com

Natural Partners, Inc.
(888) 633-7620
www.naturalpartners.com

Mia's Recommended Stress Relief Products

Healing Rhythms

A personal training tool using state of the art technology with beautiful visuals, soothing sounds, and effective meditation and breathing techniques to help you uncover your body's natural ability to counter the effects of stress.

www.wilddivine.com/

emWave

emWave Personal Stress Reliever provides a handheld, portable, and convenient way to reduce stress, balance emotions, and increase performance anytime, anywhere. It is especially useful when preparing for highly stressful meetings, for improving sleep, to improve athletic performance, to overcome the effects of stress associated with health issues, or to recover quickly from stressful situations.

emWave Personal Stress Reliever, uses drug-free stress relief technology to help you balance your emotions, mind, and body. Step-by-step, through narration, animations, and music, the Coherence Coach gives you the stress relief training to increase coherence levels while using your emWave.

www.emwave.com/

Resperate

Resperate is a portable electronic biofeedback device that can help lower blood pressure and your stress level.

www.resperate.com

Other Helpful Websites and Organizations

Thyroid Info.com

http://www.thyroid-info.com/index.htm

Patient advocate and writer Mary Shomon transformed her own 1995 thyroid diagnosis into a mission to educate and empower other patients who struggle with thyroid, autoimmune, and weight loss challenges.

Broda O. Barnes, M.D., Research Foundation, Inc.

http://www.brodabarnes.org

Sticking Out Our Neck—Thyroid Disease Email Newsletter

http://www.thyroid-info.com/newsletters.htm

If you want to be informed, empowered, and get the information you need to live well with your thyroid condition, subscribe for free to this email newsletter.

Drug Interactions Checker

http://www.drugs.com/drug_interactions.html

The Drug Interactions Checker explains the mechanism of each drug interaction, the level of significance of the interaction (major, moderate, or minor), and in certain cases can provide the recommended course of action to manage the interaction. The Drug Interactions Checker will also display any interaction between your chosen drug(s) and food.

Thyroid Drug Information Center

http://www.thyroid-info.com/drugs/index.htm

A very informative site that gives you all the information you need on all the different thyroid medications available.

Bioidentical Hormone Society

http://www.bioidenticalhormonesociety.com/index.html

National Headache Foundation

428 W St. James Place, 2nd Floor

Chicago, IL 60614

(800) 843-2256

www.headaches.org

National Osteoporosis Foundation

1150 17th Street, NW, Suite 500

Washington, DC 20036

(202) 223-2226

www.nof.org

Postpartum Support International

927 North Kellogg Avenue

Santa Barbara, CA 93111

(805) 967-7636

www.postpartum.net

Women's Health Connection
PO Box 6338
Madison, WI 53716
(800) 366-6632
www.womenshealthconnection.com

Women To Women
www.womentowomen.com

A Friend Indeed—Initiatives for Woman's Health, Inc.
P. O. Box 260
Pembina, ND 58271
www.afriendindeed.ca

American Menopause Foundation, Inc.
The Empire State Building
350 Fifth Avenue, Ste. #2822
New York, NY 10118
(212) 714-2398
www.americanmenopause.org

Connections—Women's Health Connection
P. O. Box 6338
Madison, WI 53716-0338
(800) 366-6632
www.womenshealthconnection.com

Medical Letter—John R. Lee, M.D.
c/o Publishers Management Corporation
P. O. Box 84900
Phoenix, AZ 85071
(800) 528-0559
www.johnleemd.com

References

Chapter One: Why the Female Brain Goes Insane

Abramowitz ES, Baker AH, Fleischer SF. "Onset of depressive psychiatric crises and the menstrual cycle." *Am J Psychiatry*. 1982 Apr; 139(4):475–478.

Ahonkas A, Kaukoranta J, Aito M. "Effect of estradiol on postpartum depression." *Psychopharmacology*. 1999;146:1081–10.

Asqualini C, Olivier V, Guibert B, Frain O, Leviel V. "Acute stimulatory effect of estradiol on striatal dopamine synthesis." *J Neurochem*. 1995 Oct;65(4):1651–7.

Attali G, Weizman A, Gil-Ad I, Rehavi M. "Opposite modulatory effects of ovarian hormones on rat brain dopamine and serotonin transporters." *Brain Res*. 1977;756:153–9.

Banasr M, Hery M, Brezun JM, Daszuta A. "Serotonin mediates oestrogen stimulation of cell proliferation in the adult dentate gyrus." *Eur J Neurosci*. 2001 Nov;14(9):1417–24.

Barnes N, Sharp T. "A review of central 5-HT receptors and their function." *Neuropharmacology*. 1999;38:1083–152.

Bernardi M, Vergoni A, Sandrini M, Tagliavini S, Bertolini A. "Influence of ovariectomy, estradiol and progesterone on the behavior of mice in an experimental model of depression." *Physiol Behav.* 1989;45:1067–8.

Bethea CL, Pecins-Thompson M, Schutzer W, Gundlah C, Lu Z. "Ovarian steroids and serotonin neural function." *Mol Neurobiol.* 1998;18:87–122.

Biegon A, Reches A, Snyder L, McEwen B. "Serotonergic and noradrenergic receptors in the rat brain: modulation by chronic exposure to ovarian hormones." *Life Sci.* 1983;32:2015–21.

Blum I, Lerman M, Misrachi I, Nordenberg Y, Grosskopf I, Weizman A, Levy-Schiff R, Sulkes J, Vered Y. "Lack of plasma norepinephrine cyclicity, increased estradiol during the follicular phase, and of progesterone and gonadotrophins at ovulation in women with premenstrual syndrome." *Neuropsychobiology.* 2004;50(1):10–15.

Brinton RD, Thompson RF, Foy MR, Baudry M, Wang J, Finch CE, Morgan TE, Pike CJ, Mack WJ, Stanczyk FZ, Nilsen J. "Progesterone receptors: form and function in brain." *Front Neuroendocrinol.* 2008 May;29(2):313–39. Epub 2008 Feb 23.

Cardinali D, Gómez E. "Changes in hypothalamic noradrenaline, dopamine and serotonin uptake after oestradiol administration to rats." *J Endocrinol.* 1977;73:181–2.

Chang A, Chang S. "Nongenomic steroidal modulation of high-affinity serotonin transport." *Biochem Biophys Acta.* 1999;1417:157–66.

Cryan J, Lucki I. "Antidepressant-like behavioral effects mediated by 5-hydroxytryptamine receptors." *J Pharmacol Exp Ther.* 2000;295:1120–6.

De Novaes Soares, C. "Efficacy of estradiol for the treatment of depressive disorders in perimenopausal women: a double blind randomized placebo controlled trial." *Archives of General Psychiatry.* 2001 June;58(6): 529–534.

Galea L, Wide J, Barr A. "Estradiol alleviates depressive-like symptoms in a novel animal model of post-partum depression." *Behav Brain Res.* 2001;122:1–9.

Genazzani A, Spinetti A, Gallo R, Bernardi F. "Menopause and the central nervous system: intervention options." *Maturitas.* 1999;31:103–10.

Goodnick PJ, Chaudry T, Artadi J, Arcey S. "Women's issues in mood disorders." *Expert Opin Pharmacother.* 2000 Jul;1(5):903–16. Review.

Joffe H, Cohen LS. "Estrogen, scrotonin, and mood disturbance: where is the therapeutic bridge?" *Biological Psychiatry.* 1998 Nov 1; 44(9):798–811.

Halbreich U, Endicott S, Goldstein S, Nee J. "Premenstrual changes and changes in gonadal hormones." *Acta Psychiatr Scand.* 1986;74:576–86.

Hendrick V, Altshuler L, Suri R. "Hormonal changes in the post-partum and implications for post-partum depression." *Psychosomatics.* 1998;39:93–101.

Holschneider DP, Kumazawa T, Chen K, Shih JC. "Tissue-specific effects of estrogen on monoamine oxidase A and B in the rat." *Life Sci.* 1998;63(3):155–60.

Joyce PR, Fergusson DM, Woollard G, Abbott RM, Horwood LJ, Upton J. "Urinary catecholamines and plasma hormones predict mood state in rapid cycling bipolar affective disorder." *J Affect Disord.* 1995 Apr 4;33(4):233–43.

Klaiber EL, Broverman DM, Vogel W, Peterson LG, Snyder MB. "Relationships of serum estradiol levels, menopausal duration, and mood during hormonal replacement therapy." *Psychoneuroendocrinology*. 1997 Oct;22(7):549–58.

Klerman GL, Weissman MM. "Increasing rates of depression." *JAMA*. 1989 Apr 21;261(15):2229–35. Review.

Maguire JL, Stell BM, Rafizadeh M, Mody I. "Ovarian cycle-linked changes in GABA(A) receptors mediating tonic inhibition alter seizure susceptibility and anxiety." **Nat Neurosci.** *2005 Jun; 8(6):797–804. Epub 2005 May 15.*

Miller MM et al. "Estrogen, the ovary, and the neurotransmitters: factors associated with aging." *Experimental Gerontology* 1998;33: 729–57.

Morrison MF, Kallan MJ, Have TT, Katz I, Tweedy K, Battisini M. "Lack of efficacy of estradiol for depression in postmenopausal women: a randomized, controlled trial." *Biological Psychiatry*. 2004 Feb 15; 55(4):406–12.

Oppenheim G. "Estrogen in the treatment of depression: neuropharmacological mechanisms." *Biol Psychiat*. 1983;18:721–5.

Österlund M, Hurd Y. "Estrogen receptors in the human forebrain and the relation to neuropsychiatry disorders." *Prog Neurobiol*. 2001; 64:251–67.

Rodgers J. et al. "Estrogen linked to better blood flow." Johns Hopkins Medical Center. 1994. Press release.

Rybaczyk LA, Bashaw MJ, Pathak DR, Moody SM, Gilders RM, Holzschu DL. "An overlooked connection: serotonergic mediation of estrogen-related physiology and pathology." *BMC Women's Health*. 2005 Dec 20; 5:12.

Sherwin BB, Gelfand MM. "Sex steroids and affect in the surgical menopause: a double-blind, cross-over study." *Psychoneuroendocrinology*. 1985;10(3):325–35.

Sherwin BB. "Progestogens used in menopause. Side effects, mood and quality of life." *J Reprod Med.* 1999 Feb;44(2 Suppl):227–32. Review.

Small GW. "Estrogen effects on the brain." *Journal of gender-specific medicine.* 1998;1:23–27.

Stahl S. "Basic psychopharmacology of antidepressants. Part 2: estrogen as an adjunct to antidepressant treatment." *J Clin Psychiat.* 1998b;59:15–24.

Steinberg S, Annable L, Young SN, Liyanage N. "A placebo-controlled clinical trial of L-tryptophan in premenstrual dysphoria." *Biol Psychiatry.* 1999 Feb 1;45(3):313–20.

Steiner M, Dunn E, Born L. "Hormones and mood: From menarche to menopause and beyond." *J Affect Disord.* 2003 Mar;74(1):67–83. Review.

Thomson J, Oswald I. "Effect of oestrogen on the sleep, mood, and anxiety of menopausal women." *Br Med J.* 1977 Nov 19;2(6098):1317–9.

Woods NF, Lentz MJ, Mitchell ES, Shaver J, Heitkemper M. "Luteal phase ovarian steroids, stress arousal, premenses perceived stress, and premenstrual symptoms." *Res Nurs Health.* 1998 Apr; 21(2):129–42.

Chapter Two: The Bioidentical Hormone Solution

Adams MR et al. "Inhibition of coronary artery athrosclerosis by 17-beta estradiol in ovariectomized monkeys: lack of an effect of added progesterone." *Arteriosclerosis.* 1990;10:1051–7.

Adams MR, Golden DL, Clarkson TB. "Conjugated equine estrogens alone, but not in combination with medroxyprogesterone acetate, inhibit aortic connective tissue remodeling after plasma lipid lowering in female monkeys." *Arterioscler Thromb Vasc Biol.* 1998 Jul;18(7):1164–71.

Adams MR, Register TC, Golden DL, Wagner JD, Williams JK. "Medroxyprogesterone acetate antagonizes inhibitory effects of conjugated equine estrogens on coronary artery atherosclerosis." *Arterioscler Thromb Vasc Biol.* 1997 Jan;17(1):217–21.

Bolaji II, Grimes H, Mortimer G, Tallon DF, Fottrell PF, O'Dwyer EM. "Low-dose progesterone therapy in oestrogenised postmenopausal women: effects on plasma lipids, lipoproteins and liver function parameters." *Eur J Obstet Gynecol Reprod Biol.* 1993 Jan;48(1): 61–68.

Braunsberg HA, Coldham NG, Wong W. "Hormonal therapies for breast cancer: can progestogens stimulate growth?" *Cancer Lett.* 1986 Feb;30(2):213–8.

Bulbrook RD, Swain MC, Wang DY, Hayward JL, Kumaoka S, Takatani O, Abe O, Utsunomiya J. "Breast cancer in Britain and Japan: plasma oestradiol-17beta, oestrone and progesterone, and their urinary metabolites in normal British and Japanese women." *Eur J Cancer.* 1976 Sep;12(9):725–35.

Bush TL, Barrett-Connor E, Cowan LD, Criqui MH, Wallace RB, Suchindran CM, Tyroler HA, Rifkind BM. "Cardiovascular mortality and noncontraceptive use of estrogen in women: results from the Lipid Research Clinics Program Follow-up Study." *Circulation.* 1987 Jun;75(6):1102–9.

Chang HJ, Lee TTY, et al. "Influences of percutaneous administration of estradiol and progesterone on human breast epithelial cell cycle in vivo." *Fertil Steril.* 1995;63:785–91.

Clarkson TB. "Progestogens and cardiovascular disease. A critical review." *J Reprod Med.* 1999 Feb;44(2 Suppl):180–4.

Colditz GA, Hankinson SE, Hunter DJ, Willett WC, Manson JE, Stampfer MJ, Hennekens C, Rosner B, Speizer FE. "The use of estrogens and progestins and the risk of breast cancer in postmenopausal women." *N Engl J Med.* 1995 Jun 15;332(24):1589–93.

Colditz GA, Rosner B. "Cumulative risk of breast cancer to age 70 years according to risk factor status: data from the Nurses' Health Study." *Am J Epidemiol.* 2000 Nov 15;152(10):950–64.

Colditz GA. "Hormones and breast cancer: evidence and implications for consideration of risks and benefits of hormone replacement therapy." *J Women's Health.* 1999 Apr;8(3):354–7.

Collins JA, Blake JM, Crosignani PG. "Breast cancer risk with post-menopausal hormonal treatment." Hum Reprod Update. 2005 *Nov-Dec;11(6):545–60. Epub 2005 Sep 8.*

Cowan LD, Gordis L, Tonascia JA, Jones GS. "Breast cancer incidence in women with a history of progesterone deficiency." *Am J Epidemiol.* 1981 Aug;114(2):209–17.

Ettinger, B. "Reduced mortality associated with long-term post-menopausal estrogen therapy." *Obstetrics and Gynecology.* 1996 January; 87(1):6–12.

Feeman WE. "Thrombotic stroke in an otherwise healthy middle-aged female related to the use of continuous-combined conjugated equine estrogens and medroxyprogesterone acetate." *J Gend Specif Med.* 2000 Nov-Dec; 3(8):62–64.

Fernandez E, La Vecchia C, Braga C, Talamini R, Negri E, Parazzini F, and Franceschi S. "Hormone replacement therapy and risk of colon and rectal cancer." *Cancer Epidemiology Biomarkers & Prevention.* 1998;7(4):329–33.

Fitzpatrick LA, Good A. "Micronized progesterone: clinical indications and comparison with current treatment." *Fertil Steril.* 1999 Sept; 72(3).389–97.

Fitzpatrick LA et al. "Comparison of regimens containing oral micronized progesterone of medroxyprogesterone acetate on quality of life in postmenopausal women: a cross-sectional survey." *J Women's Health Gen Based Med.* 2000 May;9(4):381–7.

Foidart JM, Colin C, Denoo X, Desreux J, Beliard A, Fournier S, de Lignieres B. "Estradiol and progesterone regulate the proliferation of human breast epithelial cells." *Fertil Steril.* 1998 May;69(5):963–9.

Formby B, Wiley TS. "Bcl-2, surviving and variant CD44 v7-v10 are down regulated and p53 is up regulated in breast cancer cells by progesterone: inhibition of cell growth and induction of apoptosis." *Mol Cell Biochem.* 1999 Dec;202(1–2):53–61.

Formby B, Wiley TS. "Progesterone inhibits growth and induces apoptosis in breast cancer cells: inverse effects on Bcl-2 and p53." *Ann Clin Lab Sci.* 1998 Nov-Dec;28(6):360–9.

Fournier A, Berrino F, Clavel-Chapelon F. "Unequal risks for breast cancer associated with different hormone replacement therapies: results from the E3N cohort study." *Breast Cancer Research and Treatment.* Vol 107, No 1, January 2008, pgs 103–111.

Fournier A, *Fabre A, Mesrine S,* Boutron-Ruault MC, *Berrino F, Clavel-Chapelon F.* "Use of different postmenopausal hormone therapies and risk of histology—and hormone receptor-defined invasive breast cancer." *J Clin Oncol.* 2008 Mar 10;26(8):1260–8.

Fournier A et al. "Breast cancer risk in relation to different types of hormone replacement therapy in the E3N-EPIC cohort." *Int J Cancer.* 2005 Apr 10;114(3):448–54.

Fournier A et al. "Unequal risks for breast cancer associated with different hormone replacement therapies: results from the E3N cohort study." *Breast Cancer Res Treat.* 2008 Jan;107(1):103–11.

Fournier A et al. "Use of different postmenopausal hormone therapies and risk of histology—and hormone receptor-defined invasive breast cancer." *J Clin Oncol.* 2008 Mar 10;26(8):1260–8.

Glass AG, Lacey JV Jr, Carreon D, Hoover RN. "Breast cancer incidence, 1980–2006: combined roles of menopausal hormone therapy, screening mammography, and estrogen receptor status." *J Natl Cancer Inst.* 2007;99:1152–61.

Godsland IF, Gangar K, Walton C, Cust MP, Whitehead MI, Wynn V, Stevenson JC. "Insulin resistance, secretion, and elimination in postmenopausal women receiving oral or transdermal hormone replacement therapy." *Metabolism.* 1993 Jul;42(7):846–53.

Gompel, A et al. "Antiestrogen action of progesterone in breast tissue." *Breast Cancer Res Treat.* 1986;8(3):179–88.

Hargrove, Osteen KG "An alternative method of hormone replacement therapy using the natural sex steroids." *Infertility and Reproductive Medical Clinics of North America.* 1995;6:563–674. Jensen J, Riis BJ, Strom V, Nilas L, Christiansen C. "Long-term effects of percutaneous estrogens and oral progesterone on serum lipoproteins in postmenopausal women." *Am J Obstet Gynecol.* 1987 Jan;156(1): 66–71.

Lee WS, Harder JA, Yoshizumi M, Lee ME, Haber E. "Progesterone inhibits arterial smooth muscle cell proliferation." *Nat Med.* 1997 Sep;3(9):1005–8.

L'Hermite M et al. "Could transdermal estradiol+progesterone be a safer postmenopausal HRT? A review." *Maturitas.* 2008;60(3): 185–201.

Minshall RD, Stanczyk FZ, Miyagawa K, Uchida B, Axthelm M, Novy M, Hermsmeyer K. "Ovarian steroid protection against coronary artery hyperreactivity in rhesus monkeys." *J Clin Endocrinol Metab.* 1998 Feb;83(2):649–59.

Miyagawa K, Rosch J, Stanczyk F, Hermsmeyer K. "Medroxyproges-terone interferes with ovarian steroid protection against coronary vasospasm." *Nat Med.* 1997 Mar;3(3):324–7.

Moorjani S, Dupont A, Labrie F, De Lignieres B, Cusan L, Dupont P, Mailloux J, Lupien PJ. "Changes in plasma lipoprotein and apolipoprotein composition in relation to oral versus percutaneous administration of estrogen alone or in cyclic association with utro-gestan in menopausal women." *J Clin Endocrinol Metab.* 1991 Aug; 73 (2):373–9.

Newham HH. "Oestrogens and atherosclerotic vascular disease: lipid factors." *Baillieres Clin Endo Metab.* 1993;7:61–93.

O'Meara ES, Rossing MA Daling JR, Elmore JG, Barlow WE, Weiss N, et al. "Hormone replacement therapy after diagnosis of breast can-cer in relation to recurrence and mortality." *J Natl Cancer Inst.* 2001 May 16;93(10):733–4.

Osborne MP, Bradlow HL, Wong GYC, Telang NT. "Upregulation of estradiol C16 alpha-hydroxylation in human breast tissue: a poten-tial biomarker of breast cancer risk." *J Natl Cancer Inst.* 1993;85:1917–20.

Otsuki M, Saito H, Xu X, Sumitani S, Kouhara H, Kishimoto T, Kasayama S. "Progesterone, but not medroxyprogesterone, inhibits vascular cell adhesion molecule-1 expression in human vascular endothelial cells." *Arterioscler Thromb Vasc Biol.* 2001 Feb; 21(2):243–8.

Ottosson UB, Johansson BG, von Schoultz B. "Subfractions of high-density lipoprotein cholesterol during estrogen replacement ther-apy: a comparison between progestogens and natural progesterone." *Am J Obstet Gynecol.* 1985 Mar 15;151(6):746–50.

Paganini-Hill A. "Estrogen replacement therapy and colorectal cancer risk in elderly women." *Dis Colon Rectum.* 1999 Oct;42(10): 1300–5.

Register TC, Adams MR, Golden DL, Clarkson TB. "Conjugated equine estrogens alone, but not in combination with medroxyprogesterone acetate, inhibit aortic connective tissue remodeling after plasma lipid lowering in female monkeys." *Athrioscler Thromb Vasc Biol.* 1998 Jul;18(7):1164–71.

Rosano GM, Webb CM, Chierchia S, Morgani GL, Gabraele M, Sarrel PM, de Ziegler D, Collins P. "Natural progesterone, but not medroxyprogesterone acetate, enhances the beneficial effect of estrogen on exercise-induced myocardial ischemia in postmenopausal women." *J Am Coll Cardiol.* 2000 Dec;36(7):2154–9.

Ross RK, Paganini-Hill A, Wan PC, Pike MC. "Effect of hormone replacement therapy on breast cancer risk: estrogen versus estrogen plus progestin." *J Natl Cancer Inst.* 2000 Feb 16;92(4):328–32.

Rossouw JE, Anderson GL, Prentice RL, et al. "Risks and benefits of estrogen plus progestin in healthy postmenopausal women: principal results from the Women's Health Initiative randomized controlled trial." *JAMA.* 2002;288:321–33

Scarabin PY, Alhenc-Gelas M, Plu-Bureau G, Taisne P, Agher R, Aiach M. "Effects of oral and transdermal estrogen/progesterone regimens on blood coagulation and fibrinolysis in postmenopausal women. A randomized controlled trial." *Arterioscler Thromb Vasc Biol.* 1997 Nov;17(11):3071–8.

Schairer C, Gail M, Byrne C, Rosenberg PS, Sturgeon SR, Brinton LA, Hoover RN. "Estrogen replacement therapy and breast cancer survival in a large screening study." *J Natl Cancer Inst.* 1999 Feb 3;91(3):264–70.

Writing Group for the PEPI Trial. "Effects of estrogen or estrogen/

progestin regimens on heart disease risk factors in postmenopausal women: the Postmenopausal Estrogen/Progestin Interventions (PEPI) Trial." *JAMA*. 1995 Jan 18;273(3):199–208.

Vongpatanasin W et al. "Differential effects of oral versus transdermal estrogen replacement therapy on C-reactive protein in postmenopausal women." *Journal of The American College of Cardiology*. 2003;41:1358–63.

Wagner JD, Martino MA, Jayo MJ, Anthony MS, Clarkson TB, Cefalu WT. "The effects of hormone replacement therapy on carbohydrate metabolism and cardiovascular risk factors in surgically postmenopausal cynomolgus monkeys." *Metabolism*. 1996 Oct; 45(10):1254–62.

Step One: Identify Your Hormonal Phase

Arpels JC. "The female brain hypoestrogenic continuum from the premenstrual syndrome to menopause: A hypothesis and review of supporting data." *Journal of Reproductive Medicine*. 1996;41(9): 633–39.

Johnson S. "Premenstrual syndrome (premenstrual tension): menstrual abnormalities and abnormal uterine bleeding." Armenian Health Network, Health.am. http://www.health.am/gyneco/more/premenstrual-syndroma-premenstrual-tension/. Accessed on 2008–01–10.

Kendler KS, Karkowski LM, Corey LA, Neale MC. "Longitudinal population-based twin study of retrospectively reported premenstrual symptoms and lifetime major depression." *Am J Psychiatry*. 1998 Sept;155(9):1234–40. PMID 9734548.

Nachtigall, LE. "The symptoms of perimenopause." *Clinical Obstetrics and Gynecology.* 1998 Dec;41(4): 921–7.

Shaver JL, Paulsen VM. "Sleep, psychological distress, and somatic symptoms in perimenopausal women." Fam Pract Res J. 1993 Dec;13(4):373–84.

Step Two: Discover Your Emotional Type

Birdsall TC. "5-Hydroxytryptophan: a clinically-effective serotonin precursor." *Altern Med Rev.* 1998 Aug;3(4):271–80.

Braverman ER, Pfeiffer CC. *The Healing Nutrients Within.* New Canaan, CT: Keats Publishing Inc., 1987.

Quillin P. *Healing Nutrients.* Chicago: Contemporary Books, 1987.

Takahashi S, Takahashi R, Masumura I, Miike A. "Measurement of 5-hydroxyindole compounds during L-5-HTP treatment in depressed patients." *Folia Psychiatr Neurol Jpn.* 1976;30(4):461–73.

Step Three: Food and Supplements to the Rescue

Bodnar LM, Simhan HN, Powers RW, Frank MP, Cooperstein E, Roberts JM. "High prevalence of vitamin D insufficiency in black and white pregnant women residing in the northern United States and their neonates." *J Nutr.* 2007;137:447–52.

Bruinsma KA, Taren DL. "Dieting, essential fatty acid intake, and depression." *Nutr Rev.* 2000 Apr;58(4):98–108.

Cartwright IJ, Pockley AG, Galloway JH, Greaves M, Preston FE. "The effects of dietary omega-3 polyunsaturated fatty acids on erythrocyte membrane phospholipids, erythrocyte deformability and blood viscosity in healthy volunteers." *Atherosclerosis.* 1985 Jun;55(3):267–81.

Cenacchi T, Bertoldin T, Farina C, Fiori MG, Crepaldi G. "Cognitive decline in the elderly: a double-blind, placebo-controlled multi-center study on efficacy of phosphatidylserine administration." *Aging* (Milan). 1993 Apr;5(2):123–33.

Ellis EF, Police RJ, Dodson LY, McKinney JS, Holt SA. "Effect of dietary n-3 fatty acids on cerebral microcirculation." *Am J Physiol*. 1992 May:262(5pt.2):H1379–86.

Emsley R, Myburgh C, Oosthuizen P, van Rensburg SJ. "Randomized, placebo-controlled study of ethyl-eicosapentaenoic acid as supplemental treatment in schizophrenia." *Am J Psychiatry*. 2002 Sep; 159(9):1596–8.

Facchinetti F et al. "Oral magnesium successfully relieves premenstrual mood changes." *Obstet Gynecol*. 1991 Aug;78:177–81.

Fontani G, Corradeschi F, Felici A, Alfatti F, Migliorini S, Lodi L. "Cognitive and physiological effects of omega-3 polyunsaturated fatty acid supplementation in healthy subjects." *Eur J Clin Invest*. 2005 Nov; 35(11):691–9.

Frasure-Smith N, Lesperance F, Julien P. "Major depression is associated with lower omega-3 fatty acid levels in patients with recent acute coronary syndromes." *Biol Psychiatry*. 2004 May 1;55(9): 891–6.

Gómez-Pinilla et al. "Brain foods: the effects of nutrients on brain function." *Nature Reviews Neuroscience*. 2008;9(7):568. DOI 10.1038/ nrn2421.

Hamilton L, Greiner R, Salem N Jr, Kim HY. "n-3 fatty acid deficiency decreases phosphatidylserine accumulation selectively in neuronal tissues." *Lipids*. 2000 Aug;35(8):863–9.

Hayley S, Poulter MO, Merali Z, Anisman H. "The pathogenesis of clinical depression: stressor- and cytokine-induced alterations of neuroplasticity." *Neuroscience*. 2005;135(3):659–78.

Hibbeln JR. "Fish consumption and major depression." *Lancet.* 1998 Apr 18;351(9110):1213.

Holub BJ. "Clinical nutrition: 4. Omega-3 fatty acids in cardiovascular care." *CMAJ.* 2002 Mar 5;166(5):608–15.

Huan M, Hamazaki K, Sun Y, et al. "Suicide attempt and n-3 fatty acid levels in red blood cells: a case control study in China." *Biol Psychiatry.* 2004 Oct 1;56(7):490–6.

Kennedy SH, Javanmard M, Vaccarino FJ. "A review of functional neuroimaging in mood disorders: positron emission tomography and depression." *Can J Psychiatry.* 1997 Jun;42(5):467–75.

Logan AC. "Omega-3 fatty acids and major depression: a primer for the mental health professional." *Lipids Health Dis.* 2004 Nov 9;3:25.

Marszalek JR, Lodish HF. "Docosahexaenoic acid, fatty acid-interacting proteins, and neuronal function: breastmilk and fish are good for you." *Annu Rev Cell Dev Biol.* 2005;21:633–57.

McCann, JC, Ames BN. "Is there convincing biological or behavioral evidence linking vitamin D deficiency to brain dysfunction?" *FASEB J.* 2008;22:982–1001. Review.

McGrath-Hanna NK, Greene DM, Tavernier RJ, Bult-Ito A. "Diet and mental health in the Arctic: is diet an important risk factor for mental health in circumpolar peoples?—a review." *Int J Circumpolar Health.* 2003 Sep;62(3):228–41.

O'Brien SM, Scott LV, Dinan TG. "Cytokines: abnormalities in major depression and implications for pharmacological treatment." *Hum Psychopharmacol.* 2004 Aug;19(6):397–403.

Peet M, Horrobin DF. "A dose-ranging study of the effects of ethyleicosapentaenoate in patients with ongoing depression despite apparently adequate treatment with standard drugs." *Arch Gen Psychiatry.* 2002 Oct;59(19):913–9.

Peet M, Stokes C. "Omega–3 fatty acids in the treatment of psychiatric disorders." *Drugs.* 2005;65(8):1051–9.

Raison CL, Capuron L, Miller AH. "Cytokines sing the blues: inflammation and the pathogenesis of depression." *Trends Immunol.* 2006 Jan;27(1):24–31.

Rubinow DR. "Treatment strategies after SSRI failure—good news and bad news." *N Engl J Med.* 2006 Mar 23;354(12):1305–7.

Schaefer M, Schwaiger M, Pich M, Lieb K, Heinz A. "Neurotransmitter changes by interferon-alpha and therapeutic implications." *Pharmacopsychiatry.* 2003 Nov;36 Supp 3:S203–6.

Sublette ME, Hibbeln JR, Galfalvy H, Oquendo MA, Mann JJ. "Omega-3 polyunsaturated essential fatty acid status as a predictor of future suicide risk." *Am J Psychiatry.* 2006 Jun;163(6):1100–2.

Thys-Jacobs S, Starkey P, Bernstein D, Tian J. "Calcium carbonate and the premenstrual syndrome: effects on premenstrual and menstrual symptoms." *American Journal of Obstetrics & Gynecology.* 1998 Aug;179(2):444–52.

Uauy R, Dangour AD. "Nutrition in brain development and aging: role of essential fatty acids." *Nutr Rev.* 2006 May;64(5Pt 2):S24–33; discussion S72–91.

Vieth R, Bischoff-Ferrari H, Boucher BJ, et al. "The urgent need to recommend an intake of vitamin D that is effective." *Am J Clin Nutr.* 2007;85:649–50.

Weissman MM, Klerman GL. "Depression: current understanding and changing trends." *Annu Rev Public Health.* 1992;13:319–39.

Young G, Conquer J. "Omega-3 fatty acids and neuropsychiatric disorders." *Reprod Nutr Dev.* 2005 Jan-Feb;45(1):1–28.

Step Four: Stress-buster and Life-improvement Techniques

Allen KM, Blascovich J, Tomaka J, Kelsey RM. "Presence of human friends and pet dogs as moderators of autonomic responses to stress in women." *Journal of Personality and Social Psychology.* 1991 Oct;61(4):582–89.

Ameling A. "Prayer: an ancient healing practice becomes new again." *Holistic Nursing Practice.* 2000 Apr;14(3):40–48.

Dayas CV, Buller KM, Crane JW, Xu Y, Day TA. "Stressor categorization: acute physical and psychological stressors elicit distinctive recruitment patterns in the amygdala and in medullary noradrenergic cell groups." *European Journal of Neuroscience.* 2001 Oct;14(7):1143–52.

Einspruch EL, Forman BD. "Observations concerning research literature on neuro-linguistic programming." *Journal of Counseling Psychology.* 1985;32(4):589–96.

Field T, Diego MA, Hernandez-Reif M, Schanberg S, Kuhn C. "Massage therapy effects on depressed pregnant women." *J Psychosom Obstet Gynaecol.* 2004;25:115–22.

Grossman P, Niemann L, Schmidt S, Walach H. "Mindfulness-based stress reduction and health benefits: a meta-analysis." *Journal of Psychosomatic Research.* 2004:57(1):35–43.

Heap M. "Neurolinguistic programming—an interim verdict." In *Hypnosis: Current Clinical, Experimental and Forensic Practices.* Ed. M. Heap. Croom Helm: London, 1988. 268–80.

Irvin JH, Domar AD, Clark C, Zuttemzeister PC, Friedman R. "The effects of relaxation response training on menopausal symptoms." *Journal of Psychosomatic Obstetrics & Gynecology.* 1996 Dec; 17(4):202–7.

Kabat-Zinn J, Massion AO, Kristeller J, Peterson LG, Fletcher KE, Pbert L, Lenderking WR, Santorelli SF. "Effectiveness of a meditation-based stress reduction program in the treatment of anxiety disorder." *Am J Psychiatry.* 1992;149:936–43.

Kuiperand Lupien SJ, McEwen BS, Gunnar MR, Heim C. "Effects of stress throughout the lifespan on the brain, behaviour and cognition." *Nat Rev Neurosci.* 2009 Jun;10(6):434–45. Epub 2009 Apr 29.

McEwen BS. "Protective and damaging effects of stress mediators." *Ann NY Acad Sci.* 1999;896:30–47.

McEwen BS. "Stressed or stressed out: what is the difference?" *J Psychiatry Neurosci.* 2005 Sep;30(5):315–8.

McEwen BS. "The neurobiology and neuroendocrinology of stress. Implications for post-traumatic stress disorder from a basic science perspective." Psychiatric Clinics of North America. *2002 Vol 25, Issue 2: pgs 469-94.*

NA, Martin RA. "Laughter and stress in daily life: relation to positive and negative affect." *Motivation and Emotion.* 1998 June;22(2):133–53.

Rizzolatti G, Fogassi L, Gallese V. "Mirrors in the Mind." *Scientific American.* 2006 Nov;30–37.

Tosey P, Mathison J. "Neuro-linguistic programming and learning theory: a response." *Curriculum Journal.* 2003;14(3):361–78.

Step Five: Adrenal Health

Bates G et al. "DHEA attenuates study induced declines in insulin sensitivity in postmenopausal women." *Ann NY Acad Sci* 1995; 774:291–3.

Bland, J. "Nutritional Endocrinology: Breakthrough Approaches for Improving Adrenal and Thyroid Function." Gig Harbor: *Metagenics,* 2002.

Bloch M et al. "Dehydroepiandrosterone treatment of midlife dysthymia." *Biol Psychiatry.* 1999;45:1533–41.

Buffington C et al. "Case report: amelioration of insulin resistance in diabetes with dehydroepiandrosterone" *Ann J Med Sci.* 1993; 306:320–4.

Casson P et al. "Oral dehydroepiandrosterone in physiologic doses modulates immune function in postmenopausal women." *Am J Obstet Gynecol* 1993;169:1536–9.

Casson P et al. "Replacement of dehydroepiandrosterone enhances T-lymphocyte insulin binding in postmenopausal women." *Fertil Steril.* 1995;63:1027–31.

Diamond P et al. "Metabolic effects of 12-month percutaneous dehydroepiandrosterone replacement therapy in postmenopausal women." *Obstetrical & Gynecological Survey.* 52(7):427–429, July 1997.

Ebeling E, Koivisto V. "Physiological importance of dehydroepiandrosterone." *Lancet.* 1994;343:1479–81.

Kalimi M et al. "Anti-glucocorticoid effects of dehydroepiandrosterone (DHEA)." *Molec Cell Biochem.* 1994;131:99–104.

Khorram O et al. "Activation of immune function by dehydroepiandrosterone (DHEA) in age-advanced men." *J. Gerontol.* 1997;52A:M1–M7.

Maggioni M, Picotti GB, Bondiolotti GP, et al. "Effects of phosphatidylserine therapy in geriatric patients with depressive disorders." *Acta Psychiatr Scand.* 1990 Mar;81(3):265–70.

Morales AJ, Nolan JJ, Nelson JC, Yen SS. "Effects of replacement dose of dehydroepiandrosterone in men and women of advancing age." *J Clin Endocrinol Metab.* 1994 Jun;78(6):1360–7.

Regelson W, Kalimi M. "Dehydroepiandrosterone (DHEA)—the

multifunctional steroid." *Ann NY Acad Sci.* 1994;719:564–75.

Schaeffer MA, Baum A. "Adrenal cortical response to stress at Three Mile Island." *Psychosomatic Medicine.* **1984**;46(3):227–37.

Yanase T, Nawata H. "DHEA and Alzheimer's Disease." In *Health Promotion and Aging.* Ed. R. Watson. Harwood Acad. Pub., 1999. 63–70.

Andrew Nierenberg, M.D., Ivor Jackson, M.D. *Clinical Endocrinology News* Volume 2, Issue 1, Page 9 (January 2007) Is T3 augmentation advisable when depression is unresponsive to other medications?

Step Six: The Thyroid Connection

Bauer M, Heinz A, Whybrow PC. "Thyroid hormones, serotonin and mood: of synergy and significance in the adult brain." *Mol Psychiatry.* 2002;7(2):140–56.

Bland J. Preface. In *Textbook of Functional Medicine.* Ed. D. Jones and S. Quinn. Gig Harbor, WA: Institute for Functional Medicine, 2005. iii.

Canaris GJ, Manowitz NR, Mayor G, Ridgway EC. "The Colorado thyroid disease prevalence study." *Arch Intern Med.* 2000;160:526–34.

Chopra IJ. "A study of extrathyroidal conversion of thyroxine (T4)to 3, 3', 5-triiodothyronine (T3) in vitro." *Endocrinology.* 1977: 101(2): 453–63.

de Benoist B, Andersson M, Egli I, Takkouche B, Allen H., eds. "Iodine status worldwide: WHO global database on iodine deficiency." Geneva: World Health Organization, 2004.

Doerge DR, Chang HC. "Inactivation of thyroid peroxidase by soy isoflavones, in vitro and in vivo." *J Chromatogr B Analyt Technol Biomed Life Sci.* 2002 Sep 25;777(1–2):269–79.

Fraser WD, Biggart EM, O'Reilly DS, Gray HW, McKillop JH, Thomson JA. "Are biochemical tests of thyroid function of any value in monitoring patients receiving thyroxine replacement?" *Br Med J (Clin*

Res Ed). 1986 Sep 27;293(6550):808–10.

Gitlin M et al. "Peripheral thyroid hormones and response to selective serotonin reuptake inhibitors." *J Psychiatry Neurosci.* 2004 Sep; 29(5):383–6.

Hertoghe T. "Thyroid diagnosis and treatment: poor reliability of the single plasma TSH-test for diagnosis of thyroid dysfunction and follow-up." *Anti-Aging Medical Therapeutics.* 2000;4:127–37.

Hertoghe T. "Thyroid diagnosis and treatment: many conditions related to age reduce the conversion of thyroxine to triiodothyronine—a rationale for prescribing preferentially a combined T3 + T4 preparation in hypothyroid adults." *Anti-Aging Medical Therapeutics.* 2000;4:138–53.

Mazer NA. "Interaction of estrogen therapy and thyroid hormone replacement in postmenopausal women." *Thyroid.* 2004;14 Suppl 1:S27–S34.

Sategna-Guidetti C et al. "Prevalence of thyroid disorders in untreated adult celiac disease patients and effect of gluten withdrawal: an Italian multicenter study." *Am J Gastroenterol.* 2001;96(3):751–7.

Sowers M et al. "Thyroid stimulating hormone (TSH) concentrations and menopausal status in women at the mid-life: SWAN." *Clin Endocrinol (Oxf.).* 2003;58(3):340–47. http://www.ncbi.nlm.nih.gov/pubmed/12608940 (accessed 2008.05.08).

Spadaccino A et al. "Celiac disease in North Italian patients with autoimmune thyroid diseases." *Autoimmunity.* 2008;41(1):116–21.

Toscano V et al. "Importance of gluten in the induction of endocrine autoantibodies and organ dysfunction in adolescent celiac patients." *Am J Gastroenterol.* 2000;95(7):1742–8.

Tsigos C, Chrousos GP. "Hypothalamic-pituitary-adrenal axis, neuroendocrine factors and stress." *J Psychosom Res.* 2002 Oct; 53(4):865–71.

Index

Page numbers followed by an *f* indicate figures.